2018–2019
HESI Live Review Workbook for the
NCLEX-PN®
EXAM

ELSEVIER

ELSEVIER

3251 Riverport Lane
St. Louis, MO 63043

2018–2019 HESI LIVE REVIEW WORKBOOK FOR THE NCLEX-PN® EXAM   ISBN: 978-0-323-52498-8

Notices

Knowledge and best practice in this field are constantly changing. As new research and experience broaden our understanding, changes in research methods, professional practices, or medical treatment may become necessary.

Practitioners and researchers must always rely on their own experience and knowledge in evaluating and using any information, methods, compounds, or experiments described herein. In using such information or methods they should be mindful of their own safety and the safety of others, including parties for whom they have a professional responsibility.

With respect to any drug or pharmaceutical products identified, readers are advised to check the most current information provided (i) on procedures featured or (ii) by the manufacturer of each product to be administered, to verify the recommended dose or formula, the method and duration of administration, and contraindications. It is the responsibility of practitioners, relying on their own experience and knowledge of their patients, to make diagnoses, to determine dosages and the best treatment for each individual patient, and to take all appropriate safety precautions.

To the fullest extent of the law, neither the Publisher nor the authors, contributors, or editors, assume any liability for any injury and/or damage to persons or property as a matter of products liability, negligence or otherwise, or from any use or operation of any methods, products, instructions, or ideas contained in the material herein.

The Publisher NCLEX®, NCLEX-RN®, and NCLEX-PN® are registered trademarks of the National Council of State Boards of Nursing, Inc.

Library of Congress Cataloging-in-Publication Data

2018–2019 HESI Live Review Workbook for the NCLEX-PN® exam / Rosemary Pine, PhD, RN- BC, Director of Education, Memorial Hermann – Texas Medical Center Houston, Texas. Former Director of HESI Live Review, Elsevier [and Fourteen others].
     pages cm
  ISBN 978-0-323-52498-8 (alk. paper)
  1. Practical nursing—Examinations, questions, etc. 2. Practical nursing—Outlines, syllabi, etc. I. Pine, Rosemary. II. Title: HESI Live Review Workbook for the NCLEX-PN® Exam.
  RT55.H48 2017
  610.7306′93076—dc23

                        2015028601

Senior Content Strategist: Jamie Blum
Senior Content Development Manager: Luke Held
Associate Content Development Specialist: Kathleen Nahm
Publishing Services Manager: Deepthi Unni
Project Manager: Radhika Sivalingam
Designer: Bridget Hoette

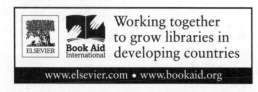

Contributors

Rosemary Pine, PhD, RN-BC
Director of Education
Memorial Hermann–Texas Medical Center
Houston, Texas
Former Director of HESI Live Review, Elsevier

E. Tina Cuellar, PhD, RN
Director, HESI Live Review
Elsevier Review Courses
Nursing and Health Professions
Houston, Texas

Lucindra Campbell-Law, PhD, ANP
Professor of Nursing
Carol and Odis Peavy School of Nursing
University of St. Thomas
Houston, Texas

Holly J. Diesel, PhD, RN
Associate Professor
Goldfarb School of Nursing at Barnes–Jewish College
St. Louis, Missouri

Claudine Dufrene, PhD, RN-BC, GNP-BC, CNE
Assistant Professor
Professor of Nursing
Carol and Odis Peavy School of Nursing
University of St. Thomas
Houston, Texas

Amber Essman, DNP, APRN, FNP-BC, CNE
Professor
Indiana University East
Richmond, Indiana

Helen Freeman, MSN, RN-BC, CNE
Consultant
Mars Hill, North Carolina

JoAnne Gaudet, MSN, RN, CCRN
Clinical Educator
Houston Methodist Hospital
Houston, Texas

Marilyn Haupt, PhD, RN
Assistant Professor of Nursing
Carol and Odis Peavy School of Nursing
University of St. Thomas
Houston, Texas

Lisa Kritz, MA, RNC-OB
Clinical Specialist
Mercy Medical Center
Dubuque, Iowa

Ann Lovric, MSN, RN
Assistant Professor
School of Nursing
University of Texas Medical Branch
Galveston, Texas

Barbara Magenheim, EdD, RN, CNE
Nursing Faculty
Chandler Gilbert Community College
Mesa, Arizona

LaDonna Northington, DNS, PNP-BC
Professor
School of Nursing
University of Mississippi Medical Center
Jackson, Mississippi

Karen O'Brien, PhD, ANP, RN
Professor of Nursing
Carol and Odis Peavy School of Nursing
University of St. Thomas
Houston, Texas

Roy Trahan, PhD, RN
Assistant Professor
School of Nursing
University of Texas Medical Branch
Galveston, Texas

The editors and publisher would like to acknowledge the following individuals for contributions to the previous editions of the book.

Diane E. Friend, MS, RN, CDONA/LTC
Assistant Professor
Allegany College of Maryland
Cumberland, Maryland

Marcia L. Gasper, EdD, RN
Associate Professor of Nursing
East Stroudsburg University
East Stroudsburg, Pennsylvania

Virginia J. Hallenbeck, DNP, RN, ACNS-BC
Clinical Nurse Specialist/Adjunct Faculty
Ohio State University Medical Center
Columbus, Ohio

Mickie Hinds, PhD, RN
Former Director, Review and Curriculum
Elsevier Review and Testing
Nursing and Health Professions
Houston, Texas

Dawn M. Johnson, DNP, RN
Program Director
Great Lakes Institute of Technology
Erie, Pennsylvania

Susan Morrison, PhD, RN
President Emerita
Elsevier Review and Testing
Nursing and Health Professions
Houston, Texas

Ainslie Nibert, PhD, RN
Associate Dean
Texas Woman's University
Houston, Texas

Judy Siefert, MSN, RN
Former Director
Nursing and Health Professions
Houston, Texas

Julia Vicente, MSN, RN, CCRN-K
Adjunct Professor
Chamberlain College of Nursing
Miramar, Florida

Denise Voyles, MN, RN
Testing Manager
Elsevier Review and Testing
Nursing and Health Professions
Houston, Texas

1 Test-Taking Strategies and Study Guide

Welcome to the HESI Live Review Course

This series of slides and the workbook provide test-taking strategies, sample test questions, and a content review of the nursing curriculum to help prepare nursing students for the NCLEX-PN examination. For a more in-depth review of certain material, please refer to the following:
- *HESI Comprehensive Review for the NCLEX-PN Examination*
- *Mosby's Comprehensive Review of Nursing for the NCLEX-PN Examination*
- *Saunders Comprehensive Review for the NCLEX-PN Examination*

Knowledge is power!

Goals of the Live Review Course
- Strengthen test-taking skills.
- Provide practice answering NCLEX-style questions.
- Incorporate recommended strategies to manage anxiety.
- Formulate a study plan using tools such as the *HESI Live Review Workbook for the NCLEX-PN Exam*.
- Review basic curriculum content.

NCLEX-PN Examination

About the NCLEX-PN Blueprint
- The test plan is revised every 3 years after a practice analysis has been conducted with entry-level nurses.
- Information about the test plan, including descriptions of content categories and related content for each category, can be found on the website for the National Council of State Boards of Nursing (https://www.ncsbn.org/index.htm).
- The NCSBN website also presents information for students, frequently asked questions, and examples of alternate formats.
- The content of the NCLEX-PN Test Plan covers essential nursing knowledge in four client needs categories.

Client Needs Categories
- Safe and Effective Care Environment
  — Coordinated Care
  — Safety and Infection Control
- Health Promotion and Maintenance
- Psychosocial Integrity
- Physiological Integrity
  — Basic Care and Comfort
  — Pharmacological Therapies
  — Reduction of Risk Potential
  — Physiological Adaptation

Processes

Processes fundamental to PN practice are integrated into all client needs categories.

- Nursing process
  - Planning and implementing nursing care based on assessment, diagnosis, and determining priorities
  - Evaluating the effectiveness of nursing care
- Caring
- Communication and documentation
- Teaching and learning
- Culture and spirituality

About Test Administration

With computerized adaptive testing (CAT), the difficulty of the exam is tailored to the candidate's ability level.

All practical/vocational nurse candidates must answer a minimum of 85 items. The maximum number of items the candidate may answer during the allotted 5-hour period is 205.

About Test Item Questions

Multiple Choice Items

- One question with four choices (answers) from which to choose the correct response

Multiple Response Items

- Require the candidate to select two or more answers from five or six choices
- The item instructs the candidate to choose all that apply.

Fill-in-the-Blank Items

- Require a candidate to type one or more numbers in a blank after a calculation is completed
- If rounding is necessary, it is performed at the end of the calculation.

Hot Spot Items

- Instruct the candidate to identify one or more areas on a picture or graphic
- Can measure knowledge related to safety, physical assessment, and other skills

Chart/Exhibit Format

- Presents the candidate with a problem that requires review of the information in the chart/exhibit to arrive at the answer
- Provides the client history, laboratory data, and clinical data on tabs

Ordered Response Items or Drag and Drop

- Require a candidate to rank order or move options to provide the correct answer
- Present the candidate with a list of the essential steps of a nursing procedure (e.g., CPR) and instruct the individual to order the steps in the correct sequence

Audio Item Format

■ The format presents the candidate with an audio clip; the individual uses headphones to listen to the clip and select the answer that applies.

■ The format evaluates the candidate's competence in certain skills or clinical problem-solving areas.

Graphic Options

■ May be used as all or part of an individual item, either in the question itself or as part of the response

Test-Taking Strategies

General Strategies

■ Every question must be answered to move to the next question, so make your best guess if you are not sure of the answer.

■ Quickly eliminate choices that do not answer the question.

■ Reread the question for qualifiers or other words that specify what the question asks.

■ Decide what makes the responses different from each other.

■ Keep in mind that the choice may contain correct information but may not answer the question.

For Your Toolbox

■ Use the ABCs of nursing (airway, breathing, and circulation) when selecting an answer or determining the order of priority.
  — Remember the order of priority: airway, breathing, and circulation.
  — An exception to the rule is, when using cardiopulmonary resuscitation (CPR), CAB is the order of priority.

■ Maslow's Hierarchy of Needs
  — Address physiological needs first, followed by safety and security needs, love and belonging needs, self-esteem needs, and self-actualization needs.
  — When a physiological need is not addressed in the question, look for the option that addresses safety.

■ Carefully read the question to determine the step of the nursing process.
  — *Data collection* questions involve gathering data.
  — *Planning* questions require collaboration and assisting with the development of a plan of care.
  — *Implementation* questions address issues of assisting with organizing and managing care and communicating nursing interventions thoroughly and accurately.
  — *Evaluation* questions focus on comparing the actual outcomes of care with the expected outcomes and on communicating and documenting findings.

■ **Think: safety, safety, SAFETY!**

■ Choose a nursing action that could prevent harm to the client.

■ Collect data before taking action when appropriate.

- Have all necessary information and take all possible relevant actions before calling the healthcare provider.
- Start with the least invasive intervention.
- Determine which client to assess first (i.e., most at risk, most physiologically unstable).
- Follow guidelines for delegating assignments. Remember the differences between the role of the licensed nurse and the role of the unlicensed assistive personnel (UAP).

The Question May Contain "Red Flag" Words

Notifying the healthcare provider (HCP) is a red flag item. Think about the appropriate nursing actions to take prior to notifying the HCP. All, nothing, never, always items are red flag words.

Practice rewording the following questions:
1. "Which response indicates to the nurse a need to reteach the client about . . ."
2. "Which prescription (order) should the nurse question?"

Common Interventions

- Small, frequent feedings
- Alternate rest with activity
- Conserve energy with any activity

Reinforce Teaching Points

- Risk factors: known modifiable versus nonmodifiable
- Prevention and wellness promotion
- New medications/self-care instructions
- Client empowerment
- Anticipatory guidance
- Incorporating client education information into the client's lifestyle, culture, spiritual beliefs, and so on

A Few Words about "Words"

Healthcare provider (HCP): The HCP is the person who prescribes care (e.g., physician, nurse practitioner).

Prescriptions: The orders that are written by licensed healthcare providers.

Unlicensed assistive personnel (UAP): These include the client care technician, nursing assistant, and nurse's aide.

Keep Memorization to a Minimum

- Growth and developmental milestones
- Death and dying stages
- Crisis intervention
- Immunizations
- Drug classifications
- Principles of teaching/learning
- Stages of pregnancy and fetal growth
- Nurse Practice Act: Standards of Practice and Delegation

Practice Rewording
1._____
2._____

Specific Strategies for Success in Answering NCLEX-PN Questions—Four Essential Steps

1. Determine whether the style of the question is

    +positive+

    or

    −negative−.

2. Find the key words in the question.
3. Rephrase the question in your own words and then answer the question.
4. Rule out options.

Determine Whether the Question Is Written in a Positive or Negative Style

- A *positive style* may ask what the nurse should do and/or the best or first action to implement.
- A *negative style* may ask what the nurse should avoid, which prescription the nurse should question, or which behavior indicates the need to reteach the client.

Find the Key Words in the Question

- Ask yourself which words or phrases provide the critical information.
- This information may be the age of the client, the setting, the timing, a set of symptoms or behaviors, or any number of other factors.
- For example, the nursing actions for a 10-year-old, 1-day postoperative client are different from those for a 70-year-old, 1-hour postoperative client.

Rephrase the Question in Your Own Words and Answer the Question

- This will help you to eliminate nonessential information in the question and to determine the correct answer.
- Ask yourself, "What is this instructor really asking?"
- Before looking at the choices, rephrase the question in your own words.
- Answer the question.

Rule Out Options

- Based on your knowledge, you can probably identify one or two options that are clearly incorrect.
- Mentally identify those options on the computer monitor.
- Then differentiate among the remaining options, considering your knowledge of the subject and related nursing principles, such as the roles of the nurse, the nursing process, the ABCs, and Maslow's Hierarchy of Needs.

A client in a skilled nursing facility reports to the PN that he has not had a bowel movement in 2 days. Which intervention should the PN implement first?

A. Instruct the UAP to offer a glass of warm prune juice at mealtimes.

B. Ask the charge nurse to request a prescription for a stool softener.

C. Assess the client's medical record to determine his normal bowel pattern.

D. Instruct a family member to offer the client fluids, up to five 8-oz glasses a day.

HESI Test Question Approach			
Positive?		YES	NO
Key Words			
Rephrase			
Rule Out Choices			
A	B	C	D

A client who has COPD is resting in a semi-Fowler's position with oxygen at 2 L/min per nasal cannula. The client develops dyspnea. What action should the PN implement first?

A. Call the healthcare provider.

B. Obtain a bedside pulse oximeter.

C. Raise the head of the bed farther.

D. Assess the client's vital signs.

HESI Test Question Approach			
Positive?		YES	NO
Key Words			
Rephrase			
Rule Out Choices			
A	B	C	D

Specific Areas of Content

Laboratory Values

Know the normal ranges for commonly used laboratory tests, what variations mean, and the *best* nursing actions.

- H & H
- WBC, RBC, platelets
- Electrolytes: K^+, Na^+, Ca^{2+}, Mg^{2+}, Cl^-, $PO_4^=$
- BUN and creatinine
- Relationship of Ca^{2+} to PO_4
- ABGs, including SaO_2
- PT, INR, PTT (don't get them confused)

A client who has hyperparathyroidism is scheduled to receive a prescribed dose of oral phosphate. The PN notes that the client's serum calcium level is 12.5 mg/dL. What action should the PN implement?

A. Hold the phosphate and notify the healthcare provider.

B. Review the client's serum parathyroid hormone level.

C. Give a PRN dose of IV calcium per protocol.

D. Administer the dose of oral phosphate.

HESI Test Question Approach			
Positive?		YES	NO
Key Words			
Rephrase			
Rule Out Choices			
A	B	C	D

In completing a client's preoperative routine, the PN finds that the operative permit has not been signed. The client begins to ask more questions about the surgical procedure. What action should the PN take next?

A. Witness the client's signature on the permit.
B. Answer the client's questions about the surgery.
C. Inform the charge nurse that the client has questions about the surgery.
D. Reassure the client that the surgeon will answer any questions before the anesthesia is administered.

HESI Test Question Approach			
Positive?		YES	NO
Key Words			
Rephrase			
Rule Out Choices			
A	B	C	D

Nutrition
- Be able to identify foods relative to their sodium content (high or low), potassium level (high or low), and high levels of phosphate, iron, or vitamin K.
- Chemotherapy, GI/GU disturbances
- Proteins, CHOs, fats
- Pregnancy and fetal growth needs
- Remember the following concepts:
  — Introducing one food at a time (infants, allergies)
  — Progression (As Tolerated)

Medication Administration and Pharmacology
Pharmacological treatment and related nursing implications are reviewed in each chapter to coincide with the disease processes and conditions of the client.

Think: Safety, *safety,* SAFETY!

Reflect on the whole picture.

Safe medication administration is more than just knowing the action of the medications. It also includes:
- The "6 rights" (six *plus* technique of skill execution)
  — Right drug
  — Right dose
  — Right route
  — Right time
  — Right patient
  — Right documentation
- Drug interactions
- Vulnerable organs ($\sqrt{}$ labs; what to assess)
- Allergies and presence of suprainfections
- Concept of peak and trough

How you would know:
— Whether the drug is working
— If a problem has arisen

Teaching: safety, empowerment, compliance

Practical Tips
Do not respond to the NCLEX question based on your personal experiences including:
- *Your* past client care experiences or agency
- A familiar phrase or term
- "Of course, *I* would have already . . ."
- What *you* think is *realistic*
- *Your* children, pregnancies, parents, elders, personal response to a drug, and so on

Do respond based on:

- The ABCs
- Scientific, behavioral, sociological principles
- Principles of teaching/learning
- Maslow's Hierarchy of Needs
- Nursing process
- What the question asks—no more and no less
- NCLEX-PN ideal hospital
- Basic A & P
- Critical thinking

Best Practice for a Successful NCLEX-PN Exam

Manage Anxiety Between Now and the Test

- Think positively and believe in yourself.
- Use positive self-talk ("I can do this!").
- Set up a study schedule and stick to it.
- Avoid negative people.
- Respect your body and your mind.
- Establish a balanced lifestyle (i.e., a regular schedule for sleeping, eating, exercising, socializing, and working).

Develop a Study Schedule

- Organize resources.
  — Online texts, hardcopy books, review questions
  — Practice tests, case studies
- Identify your strengths and challenges; review the following:
  — Results of your HESI Exit Exam
  — Final grades
  — Feedback on clinical performance
  — Results of practice tests
  — Your personal identification of your strengths and weaknesses of content during this Live Review Course (LRC)
- Initially take practice tests specific to your areas of weakness.
- Establish a study schedule that includes adequate time to prepare.
- Know your testing date.
  — Plan your schedule for the 4 to 8 weeks before your testing date.
- Would a study group help you?
- Make sure you have a comfortable level of understanding of growth and development markers, labs, drug categories, drug calculations, and immunization schedules.

A Week Before the Exam

- Take a test drive to the site.
- Be mindful of traffic patterns.
- Familiarize yourself with the test center.
- Confirm that you have all the documents you need to be admitted to the exam.

The Day Before the Test

- *Do* allow only 30 minutes to review test-taking strategies.
- If you feel the need to review your notes the night before the exam, do so, but allow for a restful 7 to 8 hours of sleep.
- *Do* assemble all necessary materials:
  — Acceptable identification
  — Admission ticket
  — Directions to testing center
  — Identification
  — Money for lunch
- *Do* something you enjoy.
- *Do* respect your body and your mind.

The Day of the Test

- Eat a healthy meal.
- *Do* allow plenty of time to get to the testing center.
- *Do* dress comfortably.
- *Do* take only your identification forms into the testing room.
- *Do* avoid distractions.
- *Do* use positive self-talk.

At the Exam

- Breathe deeply and regularly.
- Continue the positive self-talk.
- Be in the moment and take the exam without regrets.
- Do not allow the number of questions to influence your level of self-confidence.

You can do this!

2 Legal Aspects of Care and the Leadership Role of the Practical Nurse

Legal Aspects

Legal Systems
- Civil law is concerned with the protection of the client's private rights.
- Criminal law deals with the rights of individuals and society as defined by legislative laws.

  Nursing negligence is the failure to exercise the proper degree of care required by the circumstances that a reasonably prudent person would exercise under the circumstances to avoid harming others. It is a careless act of omission or commission that results in injury to another.

  Nursing malpractice is often referred to as professional negligence. It is the failure to use that degree of care that a reasonable nurse would use under the same or similar circumstances.

Malpractice is found when:
- The nurse owed a duty to the client.
- The nurse did not carry out that duty or breached that duty.
- The client was injured.
- The nurse's failure to carry out that duty caused the client's injury.

Standards of Care
- Nurses are required to follow standards of care that originate in nurse practice acts, the guidelines of professional organizations.
- Nurses are required to follow the written policies and procedures of their employer institutions.
- Nurses are responsible for performing procedures correctly and exercising professional judgment when implementing healthcare providers' prescriptions.

In the elevator the UAP overhears two nurses talking about a client who will lose her leg because of the negligence of the staff. What federal law has been violated?
A. Health Insurance Portability and Accountability Act (HIPAA)
B. Americans with Disabilities Act (ADA)
C. Nurse Practice Act (NPA)
D. Patient Self-Determination Act (PSDA)

HESI Test Question Approach		
Positive?	**YES**	**NO**
Key Words		
Rephrase		
Rule Out Choices		
A	B	C	D

The unlicensed assistive personnel (UAP) reports to the PN that a client, who had surgery 4 hours ago, has had a decrease in blood pressure (BP) from 150/80 to 110/70 in the past hour. The PN advises the UAP to check the client's dressing for excess drainage and report the findings to the charge nurse. Which factor is most important to consider when assessing the legal ramifications of this situation?

A. The parameters of the state's nurse practice act
B. The need to complete an adverse occurrence report
C. Hospital protocols regarding the frequency of assessing vital signs
D. The healthcare provider's prescription for changing the postoperative dressing

HESI Test Question Approach			
Positive?		**YES**	**NO**
Key Words			
Rephrase			
Rule Out Choices			
A	**B**	**C**	**D**

Practice Issues

- Nurses must follow the healthcare provider's prescription unless the nurse believes that it is in error, that it violates hospital policy, or that it is harmful to the client.
- If the healthcare provider confirms the prescription and the PN still believes the order is inappropriate, the nurse should contact the supervisor to intervene.
- The nurse makes a formal report explaining the refusal.
- The nurse should file an incident report (variance or occurrence) for any situation in which harm to the client may have resulted.

Advance Directives

- Assess the client's knowledge of advance directives.
- Integrate them into the client's plan of care.
- Provide the client with information about advance directives.
- Advance directives can limit life-prolonging measures when there is little or no chance of recovery.
  — Living will: A client documents his or her wishes regarding future care in the event of terminal illness.
  — Durable power of attorney for health care: A client appoints a representative (healthcare proxy) to make healthcare decisions.

Informed Consent

- It is the duty of the healthcare provider who is performing the procedure or treatment to obtain informed consent.
- The PN witnesses the signature and does not provide informed consent.
- Answers to any questions the client has about a procedure are the responsibility of the healthcare provider who will perform the procedure.

Abuse

- The National Center on Elder Abuse identifies the two most important indicators of abuse as (1) frequent, unexplained crying by the elderly individual; and (2) an older person's unexplained fear or suspicion of a particular person or persons in the home.

- The nurse has legal responsibilities with regard to reporting incidents of abuse, neglect, or violence.
- Healthcare professionals who do not report suspected abuse or neglect are liable for civil or criminal legal action.

Restraints/Safety Reminder Devices (SRDs)

- Restraints and SRDs are used to ensure the physical safety of the client or of other clients when less restrictive interventions are unsuccessful. They are used only on the written prescription of a healthcare provider.
- The nurse must follow agency policy and procedure to restrain any client.
- Documentation of the use of restraints and of follow-up assessments must detail the attempts to use less restrictive interventions.

A family member of a client who is in a Posey vest restraint (SRD) asks why the restraint was applied. How should the practical nurse respond?
A. The restraint was prescribed by the healthcare provider.
B. There are not enough staff members to keep the client safe all the time.
C. The other clients are upset when another client wanders at night.
D. The client's actions place her at high risk for harming herself.

HESI Test Question Approach			
Positive?		**YES**	**NO**
Key Words			
Rephrase			
Rule Out Choices			
A	B	C	D

Legal Aspects of Mental Health Nursing

- Admissions
  — Involuntary
  — Emergency
- Client's rights
- Competency

What nursing action has the highest priority when admitting a client to a psychiatric unit on an involuntary basis?
A. Reassure the client that the admission is only for a limited time.
B. Offer the client and family the opportunity to share their feelings about the admission.
C. Determine the behaviors that resulted in the need for admission.
D. Advise the client about the legal rights of all hospitalized clients.

HESI Test Question Approach			
Positive?		**YES**	**NO**
Key Words			
Rephrase			
Rule Out Choices			
A	B	C	D

Confidential Health Care

- All clients are protected under the Health Insurance Portability and Accountability Act of 1996 (HIPAA).
  - HIPAA sets standards for the verbal, written, and electronic exchange of private health information.
  - HIPAA establishes the client's rights to consent to the use and disclosure of health information, to inspect and copy his or her medical record, and to amend mistaken or incomplete information.

Good Samaritan Laws

- These laws protect from liability those individuals who give first aid in an emergency.
- The PN must only provide reasonable and prudent care that is consistent with his or her level of expertise.

Leadership Role of the Practical Nurse

Communication Skills

Consider the type of leadership indicated by these verbal examples:

"Do it my way."
— Aggressive communication/authoritarian leader
"Whatever, as long as you like me."
— Passive communication/laissez-faire leader
"Let's consider the options available."
— Assertive communication/democratic leader

Delegation

- The process by which responsibility and authority but not accountability are transferred to another individual
- Neither the nursing process nor any activity requiring nursing judgment may be delegated to a UAP
- Five rights of delegation
  - Right task
  - Right circumstance
  - Right person
  - Right direction/communication
  - Right supervision

Which assignment should the nurse delegate to a UAP in a long-term acute care setting? (Select all that apply.)
A. Checking the blood glucose level before meals for a client with an insulin order
B. Giving PO medications left at the bedside for the client to take after eating
C. Taking vital signs for an older client with left humerus and left tibial fractures
D. Replacing an abdominal wound dressing that has been soiled by incontinence
E. Obtaining a culture and sensitivity sample from a central line catheter site

HESI Test Question Approach				
Positive?			**YES**	**NO**
Key Words				
Rephrase				
Rule Out Choices				
A	B	C	D	E

Hand-off Communication

A communication in which important client information is shared at pertinent points of care (e.g., change of shift, transfer from one clinical setting to another)

- Ensures continuity of care and client safety
- Improves communication and appropriate delegation

A PN is preparing for change of shift. Which action by the nurse is characteristic of ineffective hand-off communication?

A. The PN tells the nurse coming on duty that a client is anxious about his pain and needs information about the use of the incentive spirometer reinforced.

B. The nurse refers to the electronic medical record (EMR) to review the client's medication administration record.

C. During rounds the nurse talks about the problem the UAP created by not performing a finger stick blood glucose test on the client.

D. Before giving the report, the nurse performs rounds on her assigned clients so that there is less likelihood of interruption during handoff.

S-BAR

S-BAR is an example of interdisciplinary communication strategy that promotes effective communication between caregivers and other members of the healthcare team, e.g., HCP, physical threapists, social workers, etc.

S (Situation): State the issue or problem.

B (Background): Provide the client's history.

A (Assessment): Give the most recent vital signs and current findings.

R (Recommendation): State what should be done.

Effective Team Communication

Communication focuses on team building, facilitating collaborating, consulting, delegating, supervising, leading, and managing.

Lateral violence refers to acts that occur between colleagues, where bullying is described as acts perpetrated by one in a higher level of authority. (ANA, 2015)

- Best practices include:
  - Use clear communication.
  - Treat others with respect.
  - Avoid gossip.
  - Rely on facts.
  - Collaborate.
  - Offer assistance.
  - Speak directly with the individual with whom one has an issue.

HESI Test Question Approach			
Positive?		YES	NO
Key Words			
Rephrase			
Rule Out Choices			
A	B	C	D

Culturally Sensitive Care

The patients' culture, religious affiliation, and country of origin influence their healthcare beliefs.

A cultural assessment answers questions regarding the primary language spoken, pain management expectations, support system, and feelings toward self-care. (For example, does the patient have feelings about the gender of the caregiver? Does the patient follow the custom of giving family members control over decisions?)

- Explain to the client and interpreter that confidentiality will be maintained.
- Use materials and teaching techniques that are culturally relevant and language appropriate.

The PN has UAPs on the team. Which client task(s) could be assigned to the UAP? (Select all that apply.)

A. Transporting a client scheduled for a STAT CT scan

B. Bathing a client receiving IV vancomycin through a peripherally inserted central catheter (PICC) line

C. Removing a Foley catheter, per the healthcare provider's prescription, and encouraging voiding in 8 hours

D. Reconnecting the prescribed negative pressure vacuum (wound VAC) to a client with a pressure ulcer

E. Clearing the alarm on the IV pump and restarting the pump

The PN is making assignments for five clients at the nursing home. The nursing team includes a licensed practical nurse (LPN) and two UAPs. Which client task(s) would be assigned to the UAPs? (Select all that apply.)

A. Administering an injection of enoxaparin sodium (Lovenox) to a client who requires anticoagulant therapy

B. Repositioning a client with a stage 3 pressure ulcer who needs a bed bath

C. Checking the residual for a client with an enteral feeding absorbing at 30 mL/hr

D. Changing the IV tubing on a client recovering from pneumonia

E. Performing a straight catheterization on a client prescribed intermittent catheterization

Which situation warrants a variance (incident) report by the PN?

A. Refusal by a client to take prescribed medication

B. Improved status before completion of the course of medication

C. An allergic reaction to a prescribed medication

D. A client received medication prescribed for another client.

HESI Test Question Approach

Positive?			YES	NO
Key Words				
Rephrase				
Rule Out Choices				
A	B	C	D	E

HESI Test Question Approach

Positive?			YES	NO
Key Words				
Rephrase				
Rule Out Choices				
A	B	C	D	E

HESI Test Question Approach

Positive?			YES	NO
Key Words				
Rephrase				
Rule Out Choices				
A	B	C	D

3 Clinical Concepts and Mechanisms of Disease for the Practical Nurse

Clinical Concepts and Mechanisms of Disease for the Practical Nurse

General Perioperative Care

Preoperative Care

Reinforce teaching:

- Diet restrictions per prescription
- Teach controlled coughing and deep breathing, incentive spirometry and/or positive expiratory pressure (PEP); activities (leg exercises, turning, mobility); use of thromboembolic deterrent stockings and sequential compression devices (SCDs); and expected outcomes and plan of care
- Review methods of pain control.
- Preprocedure verification process

Postoperative Care

- A primary goal of postoperative care is to prevent common complications.
  - Urinary retention: Check for bladder distention.
  - Pulmonary problems: Check breath sounds, O_2 saturation.
  - GI: Absent bowel sounds, decreased peristalsis, paralytic ileus
  - Monitor for infection.
  - Wound management: Wound dehiscence, wound evisceration
  - Venous thrombus embolism (VTE)

A 72-year-old client returned from surgery 6 hours ago. The client received hydromorphone 2 milligrams IV 30 minutes ago for a pain rating of 8/10. The family member requests that her father be checked immediately. On arrival to the room you find the client difficult to arouse with a respiratory rate of 6. What is the priority nursing action?

A. Elevate the head of bed and turn client to side.
B. Assist with the administration of naloxone 0.4 mg IV.
C. Assess breath sounds and neurological status.
D. Check vital signs and pulse oximetry.

HESI Test Question Approach			
Positive?		YES	NO
Key Words			
Rephrase			
Rule Out Choices			
A	B	C	D

Pain

- Pain management is client centered and can occur in all clinical settings.
- Pain is whatever the client says it is, existing whenever he or she says it does.
- Nurses have both a legal and ethical responsibility for managing patients' pain and suffering (be aware of any personal bias or misconceptions about pain management).

- Assessment includes:
  - **P:** Precipitating or palliative; **Q:** Quality; **R:** Relief measures/region (location); **S:** Severity (using a scale appropriate for age and patient condition (numerical, descriptive, FACES, Oucher); **T:** Timing (onset, duration); **U:** Effect of pain on patient.
  - Observe for nonverbal behaviors, which may indicate pain (moaning, grimacing, clenching teeth, pacing, or inactivity).
  - Assess personal cultural, spiritual, and ethical beliefs that may influence the perception of pain.
  - Special populations: palliative care, end-of-life
- Documentation includes rating before and after medication, nonpharmacological measures initiated, patient teaching performed, and breakthrough pain measures implemented.
- The WHO (World Health Organization) recommends a stepwise approach to pain management.

Nonpharmacological, Noninvasive Pain Relief Techniques

- Reposition
- Heat and cold application
- Massage therapy
- Relaxation techniques
- Guided imagery
- TENS (transcutaneous electrical nerve stimulation)

Pharmacological Types of Pain Medications

- Nonopioids for mild pain
- Opioids for moderate to severe pain
- Coanalgesic or adjuvant drugs for neuropathic pain

Nonopioid Analgesics

- Acetaminophen
- Maximum recommended dosage is 4000 mg (4 g) in 24 hours.
- Monitor liver function.
- Antidote is acetylcysteine.
- Nonsteroidal antiinflammatory drugs (NSAIDs)
  - Nonselective:
    - Salicylates (aspirin)
    - Ibuprofen (Motrin)
    - Ketorolac (Toradol)
    - Indomethacin (Indocin)
  - Selective:
    - Cyclooxygenase-2 (COX-2) inhibitors, such as celecoxib (Celebrex)

Opioid Analgesics

- Mu agonists
  - Morphine sulfate (Doloral, Kadian, M-Eslon, MS Contin), hydromorphone (Dilaudid)
  - Meperidine hydrochloride (Demerol, Pethidine)
  - Methadone hydrochloride (Metadol)
  - Levorphanol (Levo-Dromoran)
  - Fentanyl (Duragesic)

— Oxycodone hydrochloride (Percocet, Percodan, Endocet, OxyContin, OxyIR, Supeudol)
— Codeine sulfate
- Partial agonists
- Buprenorphine hydrochloride
- Butorphanol
- Nalbuphine hydrochloride (Nubain)
- Pentazocine hydrochloride (Talwin)
  Adjuvant drugs (used for neuropathic pain)
  — Anticonvulsants (nortriptyline), antidepressants (gabapentin), and anesthetics (lidocaine) are prescribed alone or in combination with opioids for neuropathic pain.
  — Corticosteroids (relieve pain associated with inflammation and bone metastasis).
- Epidural analgesics
- Patient-controlled analgesics (PCA)

Nonpharmacological Invasive Pain Relief Techniques

- Nerve blocks
- Interruption of neural pathways
- Acupuncture

Fluids and Electrolytes

Changes in osmolarity cause shifts in fluid. The osmolarity of the extracellular fluid (ECF) is almost entirely due to sodium. The osmolarity of intracellular fluid (ICF) is related to many particles, with potassium being the primary electrolyte. The pressures in the ECF and the ICF are almost identical. If either the ECF or ICF changes in concentration, fluid shifts from the area of lesser concentration to the area of greater concentration.

ECF Fluid Volume Deficit

Causes are heart failure (most common), aldosterone or glucocorticoid excess, acute or chronic oliguric renal disease, and cirrhosis. Symptoms include:
— Sudden weight gain, peripheral edema, periorbital edema, elevated blood pressure, dyspnea, and altered level of consciousness
1. Lab findings
2. Decreased hematocrit, decreased BUN below 10 mg/dL (3.6 mmol/L) (hemodilution)
Treatment:
1. diuretics, fluid restrictions, weigh daily, and monitor K^+

Fluid Volume Excess

- Causes
  — Heart failure (most common), renal failure, cirrhosis, and overhydration
- Symptoms
  — Peripheral edema, periorbital edema, elevated BP, dyspnea, and altered LOC

- Lab findings
  — ↓ BUN, ↓ Hgb, ↓ Hct, ↓ serum osmolality, ↓ urine specific gravity
- Treatment
  — Diuretics, fluid restriction; weigh daily; monitor K^+.

ECF Fluid Volume Deficit

1. Causes
   — Inadequate fluid intake
   — Loss of blood or plasma: hemorrhage, burns
   — Vomiting, diarrhea
   — Adrenal insufficiency (deficit of cortisol and aldosterone)
2. Symptoms
   — Sudden weight loss (overnight), postural hypotension, tachycardia, thready pulse, dry mucous membranes, poor skin turgor, slow vein filling, flat neck veins when supine, and dark yellow urine
3. Laboratory findings
4. Increased hematocrit; increased BUN above 25 mg/dL (8.9 mmol/L; hemoconcentration); urine specific gravity is usually above 1.030, unless renal cause.
5. Treatment
   — Strict intake and output (I & O); replace with isotonic fluids.
   — Monitor blood pressure.
   — Weigh daily.

Electrolyte Imbalances

Sodium (Skeletal Muscle Contraction, Cardiac Contraction, Nerve Impulse Transmission, and Normal Osmolarity and Volume of ECF)

- Hyponatremia (diuretics, GI fluid loss, hypotonic IV fluids, and diaphoresis)
  — $Na^+ < 135$ mmol/L (mEq/L).
  — Muscle cramps, confusion, weakness, and seizures
  — Check BP frequently.
  — Restrict fluids, cautious IV saline replacement as needed.
- Hypernatremia (water deprivation, diabetes insipidus, renal failure, and Cushing's syndrome)
  — $Na^+ > 145$ mmol/L (mEq/L).
  — Pulmonary edema, seizures, thirst, fever
  — No IVs that contain sodium
  — Restrict sodium in diet.
  — Weigh daily.

Potassium (Depolarize and Generate Action Potentials, Regulate Protein Synthesis, and Glucose Use and Storage)

- Hypokalemia (diuretics, vomiting, diarrhea, Cushing's syndrome, gastric suction)
  — $K^+ < 3.5$ mmol/L (mEq/L)
  — Rapid, thready pulse, flat T waves, fatigue, anorexia, and muscle cramps
  — IV potassium supplements
  — Encourage foods high in K^+ (bananas, oranges, spinach).

- Hyperkalemia (oliguria, acidosis, renal failure, and Addison disease)
  - $K^+ > 5.5$ mmol/L (mEq/L)
  - Tall, tented T waves, bradycardia, and muscle weakness
  - 10%–20% glucose with regular insulin
  - Kayexalate
  - Renal dialysis

Calcium (Maintaining bone strength and density, activating enzymes, allowing skeletal and cardiac muscle contraction, controlling nerve impulse transmission, and allowing blood clotting)
- Hypocalcemia (renal failure, hypoparathyroidism, malabsorption, pancreatitis, and alkalosis)
  - $Ca^{++} < 2.25$ mmol/L (< 9.0 mEq/L) + Trousseau's sign, Chvostek's sign, diarrhea, numbness, and convulsions
  - Administer calcium supplements.
  - IV calcium is given slowly.
  - Increase dietary calcium.
- Hypercalcemia (hyperparathyroidism, malignant bone disease, and excessive supplementation)
  - $Ca^{2+} > 2.75$ mmol/L (> 10.5 mEq/L)
  - Muscle weakness, constipation, nausea and vomiting (N/V), dysrhythmias, and behavioral changes
  - Limit vitamin D intake.
  - Avoid calcium-based antacids.
  - Administer calcitonin to reduce calcium.
  - Renal dialysis may be required.

Magnesium (Skeletal Muscle Contraction, Carbohydrate Metabolism, Adenosine Triphosphate [ATP] Formation, Vitamin Activation, and Cell Growth)
- Hypomagnesemia (alcoholism, malabsorption, diabetic ketoacidosis, and diuretics)
  - $Mg^{2+} < 0.65$ mmol/L (< 1.3 mEq/L)
  - Skeletal muscle weakness
  - Hyperactive deep tendon reflexes
  - Numbness and tingling
  - Painful muscle contractions
  - Decreased GI motility and nausea
- Hypermagnesemia (renal failure, adrenal insufficiency, and excess replacement)
  - $Mg^{2+} > 1.05$ mmol/L (> 2.1 mEq/L)
  - Bradycardia
  - Peripheral vasodilation
  - Hypotension
  - Prolonged PR interval with widened QRS complex decreases to absent deep tendon reflexes.

Phosphorus (Activating Vitamins and Enzymes, Forming Adenosine Triphosphate [ATP] for Energy Supplies, Assisting in Cell Growth and Metabolism, Maintaining Acid-Base Balance, and Calcium Homeostasis)
- Hypophosphatemia (alcohol withdrawal, diabetic ketoacidosis, and respiratory alkalosis)
  - $P < 0.97$ mmol/L (< 3.0 mg/dL)

— Decreased cardiac output
— Weak peripheral pulses
— Skeletal muscle weakness
- Hyperphosphatemia (renal failure, excess intake)
  — P > 1.45 mmol/L (>4.5 mg/dL)
  — Monitor for signs of hypocalcemia.

Acid Base

The basics for interpreting ABG results follow:
- pH
  — Normal = 7.35 to 7.45
  — <7.35 = acidosis
  — >7.45 = alkalosis
- Pco_2
  — Normal = 35 to 45 mm Hg
  — >45 = acidosis
  — <35 = alkalosis
- HCO_3
  — Normal = 21 to 28 mmol/L (21 to 28 mEq/L)
  — <21 = acidosis
  — >28 = alkalosis

Which laboratory result for a preoperative client would prompt the nurse to contact the healthcare provider?
A. Platelet count: 151×10^9/L (151,000/mm^3)
B. WBC count: 85×10^9/L (8500/ mm^3)
C. Serum potassium level: 2.8 mmol/L (mEq/L)
D. Urine specific gravity: 1.031

HESI Test Question Approach			
Positive?		YES	NO
Key Words			
Rephrase			
Rule Out Choices			
A	B	C	D

Arterial Blood Gas Interpretation Practice

A. Determine whether the pH value is normal, acidotic, or alkalotic.
  1. 7.31 _____
  2. 7.47 _____
  3. 7.36 _____
B. Determine whether the client is hypoventilating, hyperventilating, or has normal ventilation.
  1. $Pco_2 = 42$ _____
  2. $Pco_2 = 33$ _____
  3. $Pco_2 = 55$ _____
C. Determine whether the client is retaining or eliminating bicarbonate.
  1. $HCO_3 = 20$ _____
  2. $HCO_3 = 33$ _____
  3. $HCO_3 = 21$ _____

The PN is reviewing the electronic medical records of the assigned clients. Which client(s) is/are at high risk for a potassium deficit? (Select all that apply.)
A. The client with hyperthyroidism
B. The client with metabolic acidosis
C. The client with intestinal obstruction
D. The client receiving nasogastric suction
E. The client with watery diarrhea

HESI Test Question Approach			
Positive?		**YES**	**NO**
Key Words			
Rephrase			
Rule Out Choices			
A	B	C	D	E

The healthcare provider prescribes 3000 mL of 5% dextrose (D5W) to run over a 24-hour period. The drop factor is 10 gtt/mL. There are 300 mL remaining at 0900. What time should the PN anticipate the next bag of D5W solution to be hung? (Fill in the blank.)

The next bag of D5W solution will be hung at _____.

HESI Test Question Approach		
Positive?	**YES**	**NO**
Key Words		
Rephrase		
Math Calculation		

Safety

Sentinel Event
- An unexpected outcome involving a death or serious injury
- Accredited hospitals are expected to identify and respond to all sentinel events.
- Examples of sentinel events include wrong-site surgery, medication error, patient fall, patient death or injury in restraints, and transfusion error.

Falls
- Adult risk factors: stroke, depression, mobility issue, history of seizure, history of falls, use of assistive devices, polypharmacy, environmental issues, forgetting or ignoring mobility issues
- Pediatric risk factors: length of stay, IV or saline lock, use of antiseizure medications, acute or chronic orthopedic diagnosis, receiving physical or occupational therapy, history of falls; consider age and stage of growth and development as well.

Nursing and Collaborative Management
- Fall prevention
  — Safety surveillance
  — Assess need for pain relief, toileting, and positioning.
  — Frequent reorientation

- Client and family education
- Address environmental concerns
- Sitter

High-Alert Medications
- These are the drugs most likely to cause significant harm to the client even when used as intended.
- Anticoagulants, narcotics and opiates, insulin, chemotherapeutic drugs, and sedatives are the most common high-alert medications.
- The most common problems associated with these medications are hypotension, bleeding, hypoglycemia, delirium, lethargy, and bradycardia.
- Strategies to prevent harm:
  — Built-in redundancies
  — Double-checking
  — Smart pumps
  — Standardized or protocol order sets

Death and Grief

- Kübler-Ross's Stages of Dying
  — Denial
  — Anger
  — Bargaining
  — Depression
  — Acceptance
- The grieving process may be facilitated by therapeutic touch, displaying warm and caring behaviors, and using open-ended statements to listen and assist those who are grieving to understand their own feelings and behaviors.
- Do not take away the defense mechanism or coping mechanism the client uses in a crisis.
- Customs surrounding death and dying vary among cultures. The nurse must make every attempt to understand and accommodate the family's cultural traditions when caring for a dying client.

Infection

- The chain of infection
  1. Infectious agent: a pathogen
  2. Reservoir: where the pathogen can grow
  3. Portal of exit: exit route from the reservoir
  4. Mode of transmission: method or vehicle of transportation (e.g., exudate, feces, air droplets, hands, and needles)
  5. Portal of entry: entrance through skin, mucous lining, or mouth
- Hospital-acquired or nosocomial infections
  — Acquired as a result of exposure to a microorganism in a hospital setting

Human Immunodeficiency Virus (HIV)
Routes of Transmission
- Unprotected sexual contact
- Exposure to blood through drug-use equipment

- Perinatal transmission
- Can occur during pregnancy, at the time of delivery, or after birth through breastfeeding

Diagnosis
- Laboratory testing
- Positive result on enzyme immunoassay (EIA), formally enzyme-linked immunosorbent assay (ELISA), and confirmed with Western blot test
- An AIDS diagnosis requires that the person be HIV-positive and have a CD4+ T-cell count of less than 200 cells/mm^3 and opportunistic infection.
- Polymerase chain reaction (PCR; used with neonate)
- OraQuick In-Home HIV Test: positive result is only preliminary; must be confirmed by healthcare professional

Nursing Assessment
Symptoms
- May show flu-like symptoms in the earliest stage and advance to:
  - Fatigue, severe weight loss, swollen glands, unexplained fever, night sweats, and dry cough
  - Secondary infections
  - Cancers
  - Neurologic disease

HIV Drug Therapy
The goals of drug therapy are:
- To reduce the viral load
- To maintain or raise CD4+ T-cell counts
- To delay development of HIV-related symptoms and opportunistic diseases

Side Effects
Multiple drug interactions are possible between nucleoside reverse transcriptase inhibitors (NRTIs) and other drugs.

HIV Medications
- Nucleoside reverse transcriptase inhibitors (NRTIs; monitor for lactic acidosis)
  - Zidovudine (AZT, Retrovir)
  - Lamivudine (3TC, Epivir-HBV, and Heptovir)
  - Tenofovir disoproxil (Viread)
- Nonnucleoside reverse transcriptase inhibitors (NNRTIs; monitor liver function, reduce contraceptive effects, have many drug-drug interactions, and the names of the medications often sound-alike or look similiar)
  - Rilpivirine (Edurant)
  - Nevirapine (Viramune extended and immediate release)
  - Delavirdine (Rescriptor)
  - Efavirenz (Sustiva)
- Protease inhibitors (PIs; give with food; avoid high-fat, high-protein foods; reduce contraceptive effects; have many drug-drug interactions, and the names of the medications often sound-alike or look similiar)

- — Indinavir sulfate (Crixivan)
- — Ritonavir (Norvir)
- — Nelfinavir mesylate (Viracept)
- — Atazanavir (Reyataz)
- — Fosamprenavir (Telzir)
- ■ Fusion inhibitors
  - — Enfuvirtide (Fuzeon)
- ■ Entry inhibitor
  - — Maraviroc (Selzentry)
- ■ Multiclass combination products
  - — Efavirenz, emtricitabine, and tenofovir disoproxil (Atripla)
  - — Atazanavir sulfate and Cobicistat (Evotaz)
  - — Cobicistat and darunavir ethanolate (Prezcobix)
- ■ HIV integrase strand transfer inhibitors
  - — Elvitegravir (Vitekta)
- ■ Antiprotozoals (enhance the effects of oral hypoglycemic)
  - — Atovaquone (Mepron)
  - — Trimethoprim/sulfamethoxazole (Bactrim)
- ■ Antivirals (monitor liver function)
  - — Acyclovir sodium (Zovirax)
- ■ Antifungals (vesicants; monitor IV site closely; swish before swallowing oral form)
  - — Amphotericin B (Fungizone)

The client should have regular blood counts to track CD4+ T-cell levels and viral load.

Pediatric Nursing Considerations and Diagnostic Evaluation for HIV

Considerations
- ■ Family education focuses on transmission and control of infectious diseases.
- ■ Safety issues include appropriate storage of special medications and equipment.
- ■ Prevention is a key component of HIV education.
- ■ Aggressive pain management is essential.
- ■ Common psychosocial concerns include disclosure of the diagnosis.

Evaluation
- ■ CD4+ cell monitoring tracks progression of the disease.
- ■ For children aged 18 months and older:
  - — ELISA for HIV
  - — Western blot immunoassay
- ■ For infants younger than 18 months born to HIV+ mothers:
  - — HIV polymerase chain reaction (PCR)
- ■ The focus of nursing interventions for clients with HIV is preventing infection, promoting proper nutrition, promoting self-care, and supporting counseling efforts.

Cancer

The leading sites of primary cancer in men are the prostate, lungs, colon, and rectum. The leading sites of primary cancer in women are the breasts, lungs, colon, and rectum.
- ■ Lung cancer is the leading cause of cancer-related death in both men and women.

Primary Prevention

- Reinforce education about lifestyle changes and risk factors:
  — Smoking
  — Dietary habits
  — Ultraviolet radiation
  — Smokeless tobacco
  — Environmental and chemical carcinogens
  — Excessive alcohol use

Cancer Risk Assessment

- Genetic counseling

Health Promotion

The National Cancer Institute recommends:
- Eating at least five servings of fruits and vegetables in the daily diet
- Eating foods from protein sources such as lean meat, fish, and skinned poultry
- Choosing low-fat dairy products, including white cheese rather than yellow
- Eating whole grains
- Including beans in the diet
- Avoiding salt-cured, smoked, or nitrite-cured foods
- Limiting intake of saturated fat and added sugars

Contact the healthcare provider for any of the following warning signs:
- Changes in bowel or bladder habits
- A sore that does not heal
- Unusual bleeding or discharge
- Thickening or lump in breast or elsewhere
- Indigestion or difficulty swallowing
- Obvious change in warts or moles
- Nagging cough or hoarseness

Diagnosis of Cancer

Considerations for use in the diagnosis of cancer
- Biopsy
- Endoscope (bronchoscopy, colonoscopy)
- Diagnostic imaging (e.g., CXR, IVP)
- Radioisotope studies (bone scanning)
- CT, MRI, PET
- Ultrasound
- Laboratory evaluation used in diagnosis
  — Alkaline phosphatase blood levels (Can be elevated in liver disease or metastasis to the bone or liver.)
  — Calcitonin (May be elevated in cancer of the thyroid, breast cancer, and oat cell cancer of the lung.)

Screening Recommendations

Type Cancer	Test
Breast	BSE (early 20s; educate about the benefits and limitations); emphasis is on reporting any new breast symptoms to a health professional; CBE every three years and annually after age 40; mammography at age 40
Cervix	Pap test; HPV DNA test 21–29 every three years. Ages 30–65: every five years with both the HPV/Pap test and every three years with Pap test alone
Colorectal men and women age 50+	Fecal occult blood test (FOBT); stool DNA; flexible sigmoidoscopy every 5 years, or barium enema every 5 years, or colonoscopy every 10 years, or CT colonography every 5 years
Endometrial (women at menopause)	Report any unexpected bleeding or spotting to healthcare provider.
Lung (current or former smokers ages 55–74 in good health with at least a 30 pack/year history)	Low-dose helical CT
Prostate (men over 50+)	Digital rectal examination (DRE) and prostate-specific antigen test (PSA)
Testicular (beginning at puberty)	TSE monthly

— Carcinoembryonic antigen (CEA; may be elevated in colorectal cancer but may not be reliable due to elevations related to inflammation or smoking.)
— Tumor markers (prostate-specific antigen [PSA] for prostate cancer, CA-125 for ovarian cancer, and CA-19-9 for pancreatic or hepatobiliary cancer)
— Stool for occult blood (Do not ingest red meat, turnips, melons, aspirin, or vitamin C for 4 days before the test because this may result in a false-positive result.)

A client who is receiving chemotherapy has these CBC results: hemoglobin, 8.5 g/dL; hematocrit, 32%; and WBC count, 6500 cells/mm^3. Which meal is the best choice for this client?

A. Grilled chicken, rice, fresh fruit salad, and milk
B. Broiled steak, whole wheat rolls, spinach salad, and coffee
C. Smoked ham, mashed potatoes, applesauce, and iced tea
D. Tuna noodle casserole, garden salad, and lemonade

HESI Test Question Approach			
Positive?		YES	NO
Key Words			
Rephrase			
Rule Out Choices			
A	B	C	D

The PN is caring for a client who is 24 hours postoperative for a hemicolectomy with temporary colostomy placement. On assessment, the PN finds that the stoma is dry and dark red. Based on this finding, what action should the nurse take?

A. Notify the healthcare provider of the finding.
B. Document the finding in the client's record.
C. Replace the pouch system over the stoma.
D. Place petroleum gauze dressing on the stoma.

HESI Test Question Approach			
Positive?		YES	NO
Key Words			
Rephrase			
Rule Out Choices			
A	B	C	D

Cancer Therapies

- Surgery (May be preventative, diagnostic, curative, and palliative.)
  - Nursing considerations should include teaching specific to surgery, assessment of nutritional status, availability of support networks and possible referrals pre-op (Reach to Recovery, the Lost Chord Club, I Can Cope, Look Good, Feel Good, and local chapters of the United Ostomy Associations of America).
- External Radiation
  - Keep the skin dry. If the area becomes wet during bathing, pat the skin dry with an absorbent towel.
  - Do not apply lotions, ointments, creams, and powders in marked areas. Any lotions or creams designed to specifically manage drying skin must be prescribed by the healthcare provider.
  - Protect the radiated area from direct sunlight.
  - Avoid applications of heat or cold because these would increase erythema, drying, and pruritus of the skin, which is common over an irradiated area.
  - Encourage fluid intake (2–3 liters per day).
  - Eat a diet high in protein and calories.

Internal Radiation Therapy

Sealed radioactive materials are used (i.e., cancer of cervix). An applicator containing a radioactive material is placed in the vagina (brachytherapy).

- Special precautions
- Place Radiation in Use sign on the patient's door.
- Prevent dislodgment. Keep the patient on strict bed rest. Instruct the patient not to turn from side to side or onto the abdomen. Do not raise the head of the bed more than 45 degrees.
- Do not give a complete bed bath while the applicator is in place, and do not bathe the patient below the waist. Do not change bed linen unless it is necessary.
- Encourage the patient to do active range-of-motion (ROM) exercises with both arms, and to do mild foot and leg exercises to minimize the complications that can result from immobility. The patient also wears anti-embolic stockings (thromboembolic disease hose) or pneumatic compression boots to prevent stasis of blood in the lower extremities.
- Monitor vital signs every 4 hours and be alert for elevations in temperature, pulse, and respirations. A temperature higher than 100°F (37.7°C) should be reported to the patient's healthcare provider.
- Assess for and report any rash or skin eruption, excessive vaginal bleeding, or vaginal discharge.
- Maintain an accurate intake and output record.
- Encourage the patient to consume at least 3 L of fluid intake daily.
- An indwelling urinary catheter is placed to reduce the size of the bladder and decrease the effects of radiation on the bladder. Monitor patency of catheter. Ensure that it continues to drain well.
- Monitor the patient's dietary intake. Encourage low-residue selections to minimize peristalsis and bowel movement, which might lead to dislodgment of the applicator.
  - Check the position of the applicator every 4 hours.
  - Keep long-handled forceps and a special lead container in the patient's room for use by the radiologist, should the implant become dislodged. If an applicator or any other materials become dislodged or fall out of the patient, never touch them because the material may be radioactive. Any bed linens, dressings, or pads that have been changed for the patient must be checked with a radiation safety officer before they are removed from the patient's room.
  - After the applicator is removed, the indwelling catheter is usually removed, and a douche and enema are commonly prescribed.
  - Precautions are no longer needed after removal of the applicator. Encourage the patient to ambulate and gradually resume activities.
  - Sexual intercourse is usually delayed for 7 to 10 days.
  - Instruct the patient to notify the healthcare provider of nausea, vomiting, diarrhea, frequent or painful urination, or a temperature higher than 100°F (37.7°C).

— Unsealed internal radiation (i.e., radioactive iodine-131 [131I for thyroid cancer])
- Special precautions
  — Assign patient to a private room.
  — Limit the time spent in the patient's room. Work quickly, and enter only as necessary.
  — When in the room, maintain as much distance from the patient as possible. A few feet of distance makes a lot of difference in the amount of exposure to the nurse.
  — Wear personal protective equipment as indicated by policy.
  — Wear dosimeter when in the patient's room.
  — The patient is confined to the room.
  — Removal of trash, linen, and equipment from the room must be approved by the Radiation Safety Officer.
  — Pregnant and breastfeeding personnel will not enter the area.
  — All clothes and bed linens used by the patient should be placed in the laundry bag provided and should be left in the patient's room.
  — No housekeeping staff is allowed until the room is officially released.
  — Food is delivered only by nursing staff. It is delivered to the door and picked up by the patient. Mail, flowers, and other items are delivered in the same way.
  — Whenever possible, only disposable items may be used in the care of these patients. These items should be placed in the designated waste container.
  — If a nurse, attendant, or anyone else knows or suspects that his or her skin or clothing (including shoes) is contaminated, that person should notify the nursing supervisor immediately.

The charge nurse is assigning rooms for four new clients. Only one private room is available on the oncology unit. Which client should the PN expect to be placed in the private room?
A. The client with ovarian cancer who is receiving chemotherapy
B. The client with breast cancer who is receiving external beam radiation
C. The client with prostate cancer who has just had a transurethral resection
D. The client with cervical cancer who is receiving intracavitary radiation

HESI Test Question Approach			
Positive?		YES	NO
Key Words			
Rephrase			
Rule Out Choices			
A	B	C	D

A 20-year-old client has been receiving chemotherapy for acute lymphocytic leukemia. Which statement by the client indicates understanding of the nurse's discharge teaching about leukopenia?

A. "I'm relieved that I don't have any activity restrictions."

B. "I'd better wash my hands carefully, because my son can catch leukopenia."

C. "I should avoid close contact with people who might give me an infection."

D. "I need to be careful not to cut myself when shaving, because I may not be able to stop the bleeding."

HESI Test Question Approach			
Positive?		**YES**	**NO**
Key Words			
Rephrase			
Rule Out Choices			
A	**B**	**C**	**D**

A client who is postoperative for a colectomy complains, "I just felt a popping right after I coughed." The PN notes a large amount of serosanguineous drainage and the intestines protruding slightly from the incision. The LPN should immediately implement which priority intervention(s)? (Select all that apply.)

A. Encourage the client to turn and breathe deeply while splinting the opening.

B. Cover the wound with a moist, sterile, normal saline dressing.

C. Document the appearance of loops of bowel through the wound.

D. Reinsert the organs and apply a firm pressure dressing.

E. Place the client in a low Fowler's position with the knees bent.

F. Contact the charge nurse and call the healthcare provider.

HESI Test Question Approach					
Positive?				**YES**	**NO**
Key Words					
Rephrase					
Rule Out Choices					
A	**B**	**C**	**D**	**E**	**F**

A client expresses anxiety to the PN about an upcoming surgery. Which response by the PN is likely to be most supportive of the client?

A. "Tell me what has been shared with you about the surgery."

B. "Let me review the postoperative care you'll receive after surgery."

C. "Don't worry. Your surgeon has the best record of success."

D. "I had surgery just like that, and I'm fine."

HESI Test Question Approach			
Positive?		**YES**	**NO**
Key Words			
Rephrase			
Rule Out Choices			
A	**B**	**C**	**D**

The PN checks a client's abdominal surgical incision for signs of infection. Which sign or symptom would indicate an infection? (Select all that apply.)

A. The client refuses to cough and breathe deeply as directed.
B. The client complains of a pain level of 7 on a scale of 1 to 10.
C. A moderate amount of serosanguineous drainage is present on the gauze dressing.
D. The client complains of chills and tremors.
E. The client's vital signs are: temperature, 100.4°F (38° C); pulse, 106 beats/min; respiration, 20 breaths/min.

HESI Test Question Approach				
Positive?			YES	NO
Key Words				
Rephrase				
Rule Out Choices				
A	B	C	D	E

4 Advanced Clinical Concepts and Disaster Management

Acute Conditions

Shock

Assessment and monitoring of shock states focus on changes in pulse rate and quality as the main indicator of shock presence or progression.

Stages of Shock

- Stage 1: Initial Stage
  - MAP ↓ 10 mm Hg from baseline.
  - ↑ Heart rate
  - ↑ Respiratory rate
- Stage 2: Nonprogressive Stage
  - Restlessness
  - MAP Decrease 10–15 mm Hg from baseline
  - ↑ Heart rate (except neurogenic)
  - ↓ Urine output (oliguria)
  - Pulse oximetry 90%–95%
- Stage 3: Progressive Stage
  - Pallor/cyanosis of mucosa/nail beds
  - ↓ in MAP > 20 mm Hg
  - ↓ PH, ↑ Lactate levels
  - Rapid weak, thready pulses
  - Cool, moist skin
  - Pulse oximetry 75%–80%
  - Anuria
- Stage 4: Refractory Stage
  - Rapid LOC
  - Widespread toxic metabolite release makes patient unresponsive to shock correction
  - Slow, shallow respirations
  - Pulse oximetry < 70%
  - Multiple organ dysfunction syndrome (MODS)

Types of Shock

- Hypovolemic
- Decreased circulating volume related to internal/external blood loss or dehydration.
- Older adults risk r/t diuretic therapy, ↓thirst reflex, and anticoagulation therapy.
- Cardiogenic
  - Pump failure; myocardial infarction is the most common cause.
  - Results in ↓ cardiac output and MAP
  - Older adults risk r/t diabetes mellitus, cardiomyopathies, and cognitive impairment
- Distributive or vasogenic
  - Anaphylactic, neurogenic, and septic shock
  - Excessive vasodilation and impaired distribution of blood flow
  - Older adults risk r/t ↓immune response, malignancies, or malnutrition

- Obstructive
  - Physical obstruction that impedes the filling and pumping of the heart
  - Pericarditis or cardiac tamponade
  - Older adult risk r/t autoimmune disorders, malignancies, and pulmonary hypertension.

Best Practice for Safety and Quality of a Patient who is in shock

- Correct decreased tissue perfusion and restore cardiac output.
  - Optimize oxygenation and ventilation.
  - Fluid resuscitation
  - Correct positioning, monitoring, and RN collaboration

In cardiogenic shock, volume expanders may precipitate pulmonary edema.

Drug Therapy

- Restore cardiac function based on effect of shock on preload, afterload, and contractility.
- Replace blood volume or fluid loss.
- Administer medications.
  - Vasodilators
  - Vasoconstrictors

Collaborative and Nursing Management

- Data collection
  - Vital signs
  - Mental status
  - Urine output

An elderly client with a percutaneous gastrostomy feeding tube is admitted from a nursing home to the hospital. The client has altered mental status, dehydration, and fever. In caring for this client, the nurse should be alert to which priority condition?

A. Cardiogenic shock
B. Acute renal failure
C. Glomerulonephritis
D. Urinary tract infection

HESI Test Question Approach			
Positive?		**YES**	**NO**
Key Words			
Rephrase			
Rule Out Choices			
A	**B**	**C**	**D**

The PN receives the change of shift report about a client who is 6 hours postoperative from abdominal surgery. At the beginning of the shift vital signs were BP, 106/74; temp. 98.6°F; pulse 78 bpm; respirations, 14 breaths/min. The urine output for the previous 8-hour shift was 300 mL. Three hours into the shift, the PN suspects that the client is developing shock. What signs indicate the development of hypovolemic shock? (Select all that apply.)

A. Lethargy
B. Temp 99.0°F
C. Anxiousness
D. Respiratory rate 25 breaths/min
E. Apical pulse 92 bpm
F. Urine output is 75 mL 3 hours into shift.

HESI Test Question Approach					
Positive?				YES	NO
Key Words					
Rephrase					
Rule Out Choices					
A	B	C	D	E	F

A client is admitted to the acute care unit with stable angina. At 0700 the client is pain free, has stable vital signs, and is on 2 L NC. At 1000, the client reports chest pain 6 on scale of 1 to 10, is slightly diaphoretic and pale, BP of 100/52, and a RR 24. Which prescription will the PN implement first?

A. Increase oxygen from 21L/min to 4 L/min.
B. Monitor a rapid bolus of 0.9% saline via infusion pump.
C. Administer prescribed oral opioid for pain control.
D. Obtain a full set of vital signs including temperature.

HESI Test Question Approach			
Positive?		YES	NO
Key Words			
Rephrase			
Rule Out Choices			
A	B	C	D

The Continuum of Sepsis

Systemic inflammatory response (SIRS) is an assortment of insults, including sepsis, ischemia, infarction, and injury. Generalized inflammation occurs in organs remote from the initial insult. SIRS usually starts with an infection. Septic shock is one component of the systemic inflammatory response syndrome (SIRS).

The syndrome starts with an infection that progresses to bacteremia, then sepsis, then severe sepsis, then septic shock, and finally multiple organ dysfunction syndrome (MODS). MODS is the failure of two or more organ systems.

Nursing and Collaborative Management

- The prognosis for the client with MODS is poor.
- The most important goal is to prevent the progression of SIRS to MODS.
- The nursing role is attentive data collection and ongoing monitoring to detect early signs of organ dysfunction.
- Collaborative care focuses on:
  — Prevention strategies

- Early recognition of subtle changes in HR, systolic BP, respiratory rate, oxygen saturation, urinary output, and central nervous system changes
- Serum lactate level
- Prevention and treatment of infection
  — Blood culture before starting antibiotics
  — Broad-spectrum antibiotics within 1 to 3 hours of admission
- Maintenance of tissue oxygenation
- Nutritional and metabolic support
- Support of individual failing organs

Disseminated Intravascular Coagulation (DIC)

- DIC is a serious disorder of hemostasis resulting from overstimulation of clotting factors followed by anticlotting processes in response to disease or injury, including septicemia, obstetric complications, malignancies, tissue trauma, transfusion reactions, burns, shock, and snakebites.
- DIC may lead to uncontrollable hemorrhage.
- The d-dimer assay measures the degree of fibrinolysis (fibrin products in the blood).
- Astute, ongoing assessment is needed.
- Early detection of bleeding, both occult and overt, must be a primary goal.
  — Assess the client for signs of external and internal bleeding.
  — Be alert for manifestations of the syndrome.
- Institute of appropriate treatment measures, which can be challenging and sometimes paradoxic.
  — Heparin infusion (early in DIC, when clots are forming)
  — Blood, FFP transfusions, and cryoprecipitate

An elderly client is confused and was admitted to the hospital 4 days ago with a diagnosis of cellulitis. Current vital signs: temp. 103°F (39.6°C), HR 109, RR 37, BP 86/42. The client requires intravenous antibiotics, oxygen, and an indwelling urinary catheter. The nurse assesses the client and develops a plan of care. Which disease does the PN expect to see on the plan of care?
A. Septic shock
B. Multiple organ failure
C. Acute respiratory distress syndrome
D. Acute myocardial infarction

HESI Test Question Approach			
Positive?		YES	NO
Key Words			
Rephrase			
Rule Out Choices			
A	B	C	D

Acute Respiratory Distress Syndrome (ARDS)

- ARDS is a severe form of respiratory failure.
- ARDS is considered to be present if the client has the following:
  — Hypoxemia that does not improve with oxygen administration
  — A predisposing condition for ARDS within 48 hours of clinical manifestations

— New bilateral interstitial or alveolar infiltrates on a chest x-ray film (often called "whiteout" or "white lung")
- ARDS is marked by alveolar capillary membrane damage with subsequent leakage of fluids into the interstitial spaces and alveoli.
- As ARDS progresses, profound respiratory distress develops, requiring endotracheal intubation and positive pressure ventilation (PPV).

Nursing Assessment

- Hypoxemia
- Dyspnea
- Scattered crackles
- Increased work of breathing
- Intercostal retractions
- Respiratory acidosis (early)
- Pleural effusions
- Decreased cardiac output
- Cyanosis

Nursing and Collaborative Management

- The overall goals for a client with ARDS are
  — PaO_2 of at least 60 mmHg
  — Adequate lung ventilation to maintain normal pH
- The goals for a client recovering from ARDS are
  — PaO_2 within normal limits for age or baseline values on room air
  — $SaO_2 > 90\%$
  — Patent airway
  — Clear lungs on auscultation

Delirium

- Delirium is an acute state of confusion and difficulty concentrating.
- Common in elderly, hospitalized adults
- May indicate an impending change in condition (e.g., sepsis)
- Risk factors
  — Sleep deprivation, advanced age, or vision and hearing impairment
  — Use of opioids and/or corticosteroids
  — Drug or alcohol abuse
  — UTI, fluid, and electrolyte imbalance
  — Postoperative (unscheduled surgery), ICU, or emergent delirium

Nursing and Collaborative Management

- Prevention and early recognition (monitor neurological status).
- Protect the client from harm.
- Provide a low-stimulation environment.
- Approach the client slowly and from the front.
- Provide the appropriate level of supervision and surveillance.
- Reorient the client and communicate with simple statements.

- Consider management with neuroleptic drugs (e.g., haloperidol [Haldol]) as ordered.
- Encourage family visits and support.

A client recovering from ARDS is transferred to the acute care unit. Awake and alert, the client has residual fatigue with generalized weakness. Current vital signs: HR 83, BP 104/64, RR 18, SpO$_2$ on room air is 94%. Which intervention does the PN recognize as having the highest priority in the care of this client?
A. Ensure a diet high in protein and fruits.
B. Perform passive range of motion every 4 hours.
C. Encourage frequent coughing and deep breathing.
D. Explain the importance of using rest appropriately.

HESI Test Question Approach		
Positive?	**YES**	**NO**
Key Words		
Rephrase		
Rule Out Choices		
A	B	C	D

The PN is caring for an elderly client in a nursing home setting who has a recent diagnosis of delirium. Which action has the highest priority in the care for this client?
A. Assist the client with dressing and hygiene.
B. Maintain bed in the low position.
C. Encourage participation in social activities.
D. Talk to the patient in quiet tones.

HESI Test Question Approach		
Positive?	**YES**	**NO**
Key Words		
Rephrase		
Rule Out Choices		
A	B	C	D

Life Support

CPR and Choking Basics (Adults)
- Cardiac arrest is the most common event requiring CPR.
- CAB: chest compressions, airway, and breathing
  — High-quality chest compressions are vital.
  — Push hard and push fast.
  — Adults: 100–120 compressions/min
- In-hospital cardiac arrest
  — Initiate CPR according to BCLS guidelines.
  — Determine unresponsiveness.
  — Activate emergency response or cardiac arrest team.
  — Call for AED and/or emergency crash cart (do not leave client).
  — Initiate compressions.
    - After 30 compressions, open airway with head tilt–chin lift maneuver and ventilate with bag-valve mask (provide 2 breaths, each over 1 second).
    - Maintain compressions to breaths ratio of 30:2.

— Once the defibrillator or AED arrives, apply quick-look paddles or AED to determine whether defibrillation is necessary; defibrillate as indicated according to hospital policies and procedures.
— Resume CPR.

CPR and Choking Basics (Neonates and Children Aged 1 to 8 Years)

■ Indications for CPR in children are different from those for adults.
— Neonates and infants: hypoxia, hypoglycemia, hypothermia, acidosis, and hypercoagulability
— Children: respiratory arrest, prolonged hypoxemia secondary to respiratory insult or shock, including septic shock
■ Guidelines vary based on child's age.
— If no response occurs, call a code or cardiac arrest in order to initiate response of cardiac arrest team. Obtain AED or emergency crash cart with defibrillator.
— Check for pulse.
  • Infant <1 year: brachial pulse
  • Children 1 year to puberty: carotid or femoral
— Compressions (begin within 10 seconds)
  • *Infants* (most): Compressions cover at least one third of the anterior/posterior diameter of the chest; depth is inches in most infants.
  • *Children* (most): Compressions cover at least one third of the anterior/posterior diameter of the chest; depth is 2 inches.
  • *One rescuer*: 30 compressions to 2 breaths
  • *Two rescuers:* 15 compressions to 2 breaths
■ Deliver each breath over 1 second (avoid excess ventilation (causes gastric inflation).

For up-to-date information on FBOA and CPR, see the American Heart Association website for CPR guidelines *(http://www.heart.org/HEARTORG/)*.

The PN is caring for a client who suddenly loses consciousness. Which intervention will the PN implement first?
A. Quickly go to the nurses' station and ask the charge nurse to call a code.
B. Obtain a defibrillator from an adjacent nursing unit.
C. Call for help and initiate cardiopulmonary resuscitation (CPR).
D. Start oxygen by cannula at 10 L/min and raise the head of the bed.

HESI Test Question Approach		
Positive?	**YES**	**NO**
Key Words		
Rephrase		
Rule Out Choices		
A	B	C	D

A 59-year-old client diagnosed with a gastrointestinal bleed is found by the PN slumped in the chair. Place the PN's actions in order of priority for this client from first to last priority.

A. Activate the code team and obtain a defibrillator.
B. Determine unresponsiveness.
C. Use the quick-look paddles to determine rhythm.
D. Check for carotid pulse.
E. Open airway and give two rescue breaths by bag-valve mask.
F. Move the client to a flat position in bed.
G. Begin compressions.

HESI Test Question Approach						
Positive?				YES		NO
Key Words						
Rephrase						
Rule Out Choices						
A	B	C	D	E	F	G

Disaster Management

- The nurse is an active team member in the event of biological, chemical, radioactive, mass trauma, or natural disasters.
- The nurse plays a role at all three levels of disaster management (primary, secondary, tertiary).

Preparedness ... Response ... Recovery

- Levels of prevention in disaster management
  - Primary: planning, training, educating personnel and the public
  - Secondary: triage, treatment, and shelter supervision
  - Tertiary: follow-up, recovery assistance, and prevention of future disasters

Bioterrorism

- Review exposure information, assessment findings, and treatment for various agents.
- Questions may deal with disasters and bioterrorism as they affect the individual victims, families, and the community.

anthrax
smallpox - usually airborne

5 Oxygenation, Ventilation, Transportation, and Perfusion

41. A client who is 1 day postoperative after a left pneumonectomy is lying on his right side with the head of bed (HOB) elevated 10 degrees. The PN assesses his respiratory rate at 32 breaths/min. What action should the nurse take first?
A. Elevate the head of the bed.
B. Assist the client into the supine position.
C. Measure the O_2 saturation.
D. Administer PRN morphine IV.

HESI Test Question Approach		
Positive?	YES	NO
Key Words		
Rephrase		
Rule Out Choices		
A	B	C	D

Principles of Chest Tube: Water or Dry Seal Management

- Chest tubes are inserted into the pleural space to remove air and fluid and to allow the lung to re-expand.
- There are three compartments or chambers to a chest collection drainage system.
  — Collection chamber
    • Collects air and fluid from the pleural or mediastinal space.
    • Fluid remains; air is vented to the second compartment, or water seal chamber.
  — Water seal chamber *doctor*
    • Contains 2 cm of water, which prevents backflow and acts as a one-way valve.
    • Shows *tidaling,* or water level fluctuations; fluid should move upward with each inspiration and downward with each expiration.
  — Suction control chamber *doctor*
    • Water suction uses 20 cm of water to aid in draining air or fluid from the chest.
    • Dry suction provides a safe and effective level of vacuum by continuously balancing the forces of suction and atmosphere.

Nursing and Collaborative Management
- Keep all tubing coiled loosely below chest level with connections tight and taped.
- Monitor the fluid drainage; mark the time of measurement and the fluid level. Notify RN if >70 mL/hr drainage.
- Observe for continuous air bubbling in the water seal chamber. This is associated with an air leak.
- Replace the unit when full.

- Do not clamp chest tube. If the chest tube becomes dislodged, cover the area with a dry, sterile dressing. If an air leak is noted, tape the dressing on three sides only; this allows air to escape and prevents the formation of a tension pneumothorax. Notify the RN immediately. Continue to monitor the client.

The husband of a 94-year-old woman tells the clinic PN that his wife has become increasingly confused over the past few days and has developed a cough. Which action should the nurse perform first?
A. Measure jugular vein distention.
B. Check skin turgor.
C. Obtain oxygen saturation.
D. Check pupillary response to light.

HESI Test Question Approach			
Positive?		**YES**	**NO**
Key Words			
Rephrase			
Rule Out Choices			
A	**B**	**C**	**D**

Pneumonia

Pathophysiology
- Results in inflammation of lung tissue causing consolidation of exudate.
- Etiology
  - Bacterial (gram-negative is the most severe), viral, fungal (rare), mycoplasma, or aspiration.
  - Community acquired (CAP) or hospital acquired (HAP)
  - Ventilator-associated pneumonia (VAP)
- Risk factors
  - Age >65 years or residents in long-term care
  - Recent surgery (abdominal, thoracic)
  - Altered consciousness: alcoholism, head injury, seizures, anesthesia, drug overdose, and cerebrovascular accident (CVA)
  - Bed rest and prolonged immobility
- Complications
  - Sepsis
  - Acute respiratory distress syndrome
  - Pleural effusion, empyema, pleurisy, or lung abscess
- Prevention
  - Pneumococcal conjugate vaccine (PCV13) is recommended for all children under five and all adults > 65 years or older.

Pneumococcal polysaccharide vaccine (PPSV23) recommended for at-risk patients (immunocompromised) 2 through 64 years old, all patients >65 years, and smokers ages 19–64.
  - Annual flu vaccine
- VAP practice bundles
  - Meticulous hand hygiene
  - Closed ventilator system and suction
  - HOB elevation 30 to 45 degrees

— Oral care prior to intubation and routinely (q 2 hours) per facility protocol (chlorhexidine)
— Drain all water that collects in the ventilator tubing.
— Suction only as needed with aseptic technique.

Nursing Assessment

- Tachypnea
- Abrupt onset of fever
- Dyspnea
- Cyanosis
- Confusion and/or restlessness
- Crackles, decreased breath sounds

Nursing and Collaborative Management

- Monitor oxygen saturation and administer oxygen as appropriate (humidified to loosen secretions).
- Teach coughing, turning, and deep breathing techniques.
- Bronchial hygiene: *Encourage use of incentive spirometry.*
- Isolation as prescribed
- Administer and encourage fluids if not contraindicated.
- Administer antipyretics.
- Manage pain.

Antiinfective Medications

- Penicillins
  — Semisynthetic penicillins (oxacillin)
  — Antipseudomonal penicillins (piperacillin sodium [Pipracil])
- Tetracyclines (doxycycline hyclate [Vibramycin])
- Aminoglycosides (gentamicin sulfate [Garamycin])
- Cephalosporins (ceftriaxone sodium [Rocephin])
- Macrolides (clarithromycin [Biaxin])
- Fluoroquinolones (ciprofloxacin [Cipro])

Chronic Airflow Limitation (CAL)

- Asthma is a reversible disease.
- Chronic obstructive pulmonary disease (COPD) is a chronic, progressive disease.
- Emphysema
- Chronic bronchitis

COPD Etiology/Precipitating Factors

- Cigarette smoking
- Environmental and/or occupational exposure
- Genetic predisposition (alpha-1 antitrypsin deficiency)

Chronic Bronchitis

- Pathophysiology
  — Chronic sputum with cough production on a daily basis for a minimum of 3 months per year
  — Chronic hypoxemia
  — Increase in mucus production
  — Increase in bronchial wall thickness (obstructs air flow)
  — Exacerbations usually due to infection
  — $\uparrow$ CO_2 retention and/or acidemia
  — Reduced responsiveness of respiratory center to hypoxemic stimuli

Emphysema

- Abnormal enlargement of the air spaces distal to the terminal alveolar walls
- Increased dyspnea/work of breathing
- Reduced gas exchange surface area
- Increased air trapping (increased anterior/posterior diameter)
- Decreased capillary network
- Increased work, increased O_2 consumption

COPD Assessment Data

- Inspection
  — Bronchitis
- Right-sided heart failure
- Cyanosis
- Distended neck veins
  — Emphysema
- Noncyanotic
- Thin appearance
- Pursed-lip breathing
- Auscultation
  — Bronchitis
- Crackles
- Rhonchi
- Expiratory wheezes
  — Emphysema
- Distant breath sounds
- Quiet breath sounds
- Wheezes

COPD Nursing and Collaborative Management

- Goals for O_2 therapy—keep the SaO_2 greater than 90% during rest, sleep, and exertion, or the PaO_2 greater than 60 mm Hg
- Long-term continuous (more than 15 hr/day) O_2 therapy (LTOT): increased survival, increased exercise tolerance, and mental status in hypoxemic clients
- Infection control techniques include handwashing, oral care several times a day, and changing cannulas. Monitor for signs and symptoms (S/S) of fluid overload.
- Baseline ABGs
- Teach the client pursed-lip breathing and Huff coughing, and perform chest physiotherapy techniques.
- Orthopneic position

Reactive Airway Disease

Asthma

Inflammatory disorder of the airways characterized by an exaggerated bronchoconstrictor response to a wide variety of stimuli

- Allergens
- Environmental irritants
- Cold air
- Exercise
- β-blockers
- Respiratory infection
- Emotional stress
- Reflux esophagitis

Drug Therapy for COPD and Asthma Medications' Goal

- Quick relief Medications'
- Long-term control medications

COPD Medication Goals

- Reduce exacerbations
- LABAs or ICSs all reduce COPD exacerbations

Bronchodilators

- Short-acting inhaled β_2-adrenergic agonists
- Long-acting inhaled β_2-adrenergic agonists
- Long-acting oral β_2-adrenergic agonists
- Anticholinergics (inhaled)

β_2-Adrenergic Agonists

Inhaled: Short Acting

- Metaproterenol: nebulizer, oral tablets, elixir, and metered-dose inhaler (MDI)
- Salbutamol sulfate (Albuterol, Proventil, and Ventolin HFA): nebulizer, MDI, oral tablets, and Rotahaler
- Levalbuterol (Xopenex and Xopenex HFA): nebulizer and MDI
- Terbutaline (Brethine): oral tablets, nebulizer, subcutaneous, and MDI

Inhaled: Long Acting

- Salmeterol Xinafoate (Serevent): dry powder inhaler (DPI)
- Formoterol fumarate (Foradil): DPI

Immediate Acting

- Epinephrine hydrochloride (adrenalin chloride [1:1000]): subcutaneous

Corticosteroids

- Hydrocortisone (Solu-Cortef): IV
- Methylprednisolone (Solu-Medrol): IV
- Prednisone: oral
- Beclomethasone dipropionate (Gen-Beclo AQ Vanceril, Beclomethasone (Gen-Beclo AQ), Vanceril, and Qvar): inhaler
- Triamcinolone acetonide (Nasacort AQ Azmacort): inhaler
- Fluticasone propionate (Flonase, Flovent HFA, and Flovent Diskus): inhaler
- Budesonide (Pulmicort Turbuhaler, Pulmicort Nebuamp, Rhinocort Aqua, and Rhinocort Turbuhaler): inhaler
- Mometasone furoate monohydrate (Nasonex): inhaler

Anticholinergics

- Short-acting ipratropium bromide (Atrovent): nebulizer and MDI
- Long-acting tiotropium (Spiriva): DPI

IgE Antagonist

- Omalizumab (Xolair): subcutaneous injection

Leukotriene Modifiers
- Leukotriene receptor blockers
- Zafirlukast (Accolate) oral tablets
- Montelukast sodium (Singulair) oral tablets, chewable tablets, and oral granules
- Leukotriene inhibitor
- Zileuton (Zyflo) oral tablets

Combination Agents
- Ipratropium and salbutamol (Combivent): MDI and nebulizer
- Fluticasone propionate/salmeterol (Advair Diskus): DPI

Nursing Assessment
- Dyspnea, wheezing, and chest tightness
- Assess precipitating factors.
- Medication history

Nursing and Collaborative Management
- Monitor respirations and assess breath sounds.
- Monitor oxygen saturation.
- Monitor work of breathing.
- Monitor mental status.
- Chest physiotherapy
- Assess peripheral pulses and warmth and color of extremities.
- Position for maximum ventilation.
- Encourage slow, pursed-lip breathing.
- Administer humidified oxygen therapy.
- Provide education on peak-flow meter monitoring, importance of medication compliance, and trigger avoidance.

The PN on the subacute unit is assigned to care for the stable ventilator-dependent tracheostomy client. Which nursing actions are most essential in reducing the client's risk for ventilator-associated pneumonia (VAP)? (Select all that apply.)

A. Administer the influenza vaccine.
B. Perform chlorhexidine oral care every 2 hours.
C. Elevate the head of the bed to 45 degrees.
D. Perform suction with only 5 mL of saline. — RT
E. Monitor SaO$_2$ every 4 hours. — not stable enough

HESI Test Question Approach				
Positive?			YES	NO
Key Words				
Rephrase				
Rule Out Choices				
A	B	C	D	E

The nurse is preparing to administer a Mantoux (PPD) for a client entering nursing school. Which action is of highest priority?
A. Prepare 0.1 solution per tuberculin syringe.
B. Assess the skin condition on the forearm.
C. Inquire about BCG vaccine history.
D. Explain implications of positive findings.

HESI Test Question Approach			
Positive?		YES	NO
Key Words			
Rephrase			
Rule Out Choices			
A	B	C	D

Pulmonary Tuberculosis (TB)

TB is a communicable lung disease caused by the bacillus *Mycobacterium tuberculosis* or the tubercle bacillus, an acid-fast organism that is spread by airborne transmission.

Resurgence of TB
- Related to immunocompromised states
- Multidrug-resistant TB (MDR-TB)

Nursing Assessment
- Low-grade fever
- Pallor
- Chills
- Night sweats
- Fatigability
- Anorexia
- Weight loss
- Dullness to percussion
- Crackles

Nursing and Collaborative Management
- Airborne precautions and/or isolation
- Single-occupancy room with negative pressure and air-flow of 6 to 12 exchanges per hour
- Diagnosis: acid amplification test (NAAT; *Quanti-FERON-TB Gold or purified protein derivative [ppd]*)
- Wear high-efficiency particulate air (HEPA) masks.
- Teach client to cover the nose and mouth with paper tissues whenever coughing, sneezing, or producing sputum. Sputum specimens are collected at 2- to 4-week intervals with a return to work after third negative consecutive sputum is achieved.
- Emphasize careful handwashing after handling sputum and soiled tissues.
- If client needs to be out of the negative-pressure room, he or she must wear a standard isolation mask to prevent exposure to others.
- Combination medication regimen
  - First-line therapy: Isoniazid (INH), rifampin, and pyrazinamide are added for the first 2 months. This therapy shortens length of treatment to 6 months.
  - Isoniazid (INH therapy)

— Pyridoxine (vitamin B_6)

— Rifampin (Rifadin, Rofact)

— Pyrazinamide

- With or without streptomycin and ethambutol

— Take as prescribed for 6 to 12 months or as long as 24 months for MDR.

— Teach client medication side effects.

TB Drugs and Side Effects

First-Line Drugs

First-line drugs are bacteriocidal against rapidly dividing cells and/or against semidormant bacteria.

- Isoniazid (INH): clinical hepatitis, fulminant hepatitis, and peripheral neurotoxicity
- Rifampin (Rifadin, Rofact): cutaneous reactions; GI disturbance (nausea, anorexia, and abdominal pain); flu-like syndrome; hepatotoxicity; immunological reactions; and orange discoloration of bodily fluids (sputum, urine, sweat, and tears)
- Ethambutol hydrochloride: retrobulbar neuritis (decreased red-green color discrimination), skin rash
- Rifabutin (Mycobutin): hematologic toxicity, GI symptoms, polyarthralgias, pseudojaundice, orange discoloration of bodily fluids
- Pyrazinamide (PZA): hepatotoxicity, GI symptoms (nausea, vomiting), polyarthralgias, skin rash, hyperuricemia, and dermatitis

Second-Line Drugs

Second-line drugs are bactericidal, bacteriostatic, and/or inhibit cell wall synthesis.

- Cycloserine (Seromycin): CNS effects. Given with pyridoxine to prevent neurotoxic effects.
- Ethionamide (Trecator): hepatotoxicity; neurotoxicity; GI effects (metallic taste, nausea, and vomiting); and endocrine effects (hypothyroidism, impotence)
- Streptomycin sulfate: ototoxicity, neurotoxicity, and nephrotoxicity
- Amikacin sulfate and kanamycin: ototoxicity, nephrotoxicity
- Para-aminosalicylic acid (PAS): hepatotoxicity, GI distress, malabsorption syndrome, coagulopathy
- Fluoroquinolones (levofloxacin [Levaquin], moxifloxacin hydrochloride [Avelox, Vigamox], and gatifloxacin [Tequin]): GI disturbances, neurological effects (dizziness, headaches), and rash

| Pulmonary Embolus (PE)

Any substance can cause an embolism. Typically a blood clot enters the venous circulation and lodges in the pulmonary vasculature.

Risk Factors for Venous Thromboembolism Leading to PE

- Prolonged immobility
- Central venous catheters
- Surgery
- Obesity

- Advancing age
- Conditions that increase blood clotting
- History of thromboembolism
- Smoking, birth control pills (BCP), and pregnancy

Signs and Symptoms
- Dyspnea, tachypnea, tachycardia, and chest pain
- Apprehension, restlessness, and a feeling of impending doom
- Cough, hemoptysis, and diaphoresis
- Crackles, pleural friction rub
- Decreased arterial oxygen saturation (SaO_2), respiratory alkalosis, then respiratory acidosis
- Diagnosed by physical findings, computed tomography (CT), and transesophageal echocardiography (TEE) results

Nursing and Collaborative Management
Prevention
- Range-of-motion exercises
- Ambulate and turn.
- Use antiembolism and pneumatic compression stockings.
- Assess peripheral circulation.
- Administer prescribed prophylactic low-dose anticoagulant and antiplatelet drugs.
- Teach the client and family about precautions.
- Encourage smoking cessation.

Acute Management
- Oxygen therapy
- Monitor blood gases (ABGs) and pulse oximetry.
- Check vital signs, lung sounds, and cardiac and respiratory status.
- Anticoagulants prevent embolus enlargement and prevent new clots from forming. Used with caution in a client with active bleeding, stroke, and recent trauma or surgery.
- Heparin is typically used unless the PE is massive or occurs with hemodynamic instability.
- Alteplase (Activase, tPA), fibrinolytic drug
- Therapeutic PTT values usually range from 1.5 to 2.5 times the normal range.
- Both heparin and fibrinolytic drugs are high-alert drugs.
- Embolectomy
- Inferior vena cava filtration with placement of a vena cava filter

Hematological Problems

Anemia
- Iron deficiency anemia
- Thalassemias (decreased globin synthesis)
- Cobalamin (vitamin B_{12}) deficiency
- Folic acid deficiency
- Aplastic anemia
- Anemia of myeloproliferative diseases (e.g., leukemia) and myelodysplasia
- Chronic diseases or disorders

WBC
RBC
Platelets
H + H

- Chemotherapy
- Blood loss
- Chronic gastritis
- Menstrual flow
- Hemorrhoids

Nursing Assessment

- Pallor
- Fatigue
- Exercise intolerance
- Tachycardia
- Dyspnea
- Risk factors
- Diet low in iron, vitamin B_{12} deficiency, history of bleeding, and long-term NSAID use
- Hgb < 100 mmol/L (10 g/dL), Hct < 0.36 volume fraction (36%), RBCs $< 4 \times 10^{12}$/L

Nursing and Collaborative Management

- Treatment of underlying pathology
- Encourage diet high in iron-rich foods, folic acid, vitamin B_{12}, vitamin B_6, amino acids, and vitamin C.
- Give parenteral iron via Z-track technique.

Hypertension (HTN)

- Persistent BP elevation $> 140/90$ mmHg
- Risk factors
- Nonmodifiable: family history, gender, age, and ethnicity
- Modifiable: use of alcohol, tobacco, caffeine; sedentary lifestyle; and obesity

Medications

- Diuretics
  — Thiazides, metolazone (Zaroxolyn)
- Antihypertensive
  — Prazosin hydrochloride (Minipress), atenolol (Tenormin), and clonidine (Catapres)
- ACE inhibitors
  — Lisinopril
- Calcium channel blockers
  — Diltiazem hydrochloride (Cardizem)

HTN Education

- The number one cause of stroke (cerebrovascular accident [CVA]) is noncompliance with HTN medications.

Coronary Artery Disease (CAD)

- Prevalent etiologies of CAD
  — Atherosclerosis: partially or completely blocked coronary arteries
  — Coronary vasospasm
  — Microvascular angina
- CAD results in ischemia and infarction of myocardial tissue.
- Left anterior descending artery (LAD) is most commonly affected.
- CAD is the number one health problem in the United States.

Client Education

- Risk factor reduction
  — Smoking cessation
  — Weight reduction
  — DASH diet
  — Increase physical activity
  — Stress reduction
- Medication compliance: antihypertensive, anti-lipidemics

Angina

- Stable angina: predictable, subsides with rest.
- Unstable angina: unpredictable, may not subside with rest or nitroglycerin.
- It may radiate to either arm and to shoulder, jaw, neck, or epigastric area.
- *Other S/S:* dyspnea, tachycardia, palpitations, nausea and vomiting, dyspepsia, fatigue, diaphoresis, pallor, and syncope
- It is often precipitated by exercise, exposure to cold, a heavy meal, stress, and intercourse.

Diet Therapy

- Dietary modification: DASH
- Goal is to reduce serum cholesterol and serum triglycerides.
- Maintain ideal body weight.
- Daily cholesterol intake should be restricted to <200 mg/day.

Drug Classes for Angina, MI, or CAD Management

- Antiplatelet agents
  — Acetylsalicylic acid (ASA, aspirin)
  — Clopidogrel (Plavix)
  — GPIIb/IIIa inhibitor eptifibatide (Integrilin)
- β-blockers: first-line agents
  — Atenolol (Tenormin)
  — Metoprolol tartrate (Lopressor, Betaloc)
- Nitrates
  — Nitroglycerin
  — Isosorbide dinitrate
  — Sodium nitroprusside
- Calcium channel blockers
  — Diltiazem (Cardizem)
  — Verapamil hydrochloride (Calan)
- Thrombolytics
  — Alteplase (recombinant t-PA [Activase, Cathflo])
  — Streptokinase (SK, Streptase)
- Anticoagulants
  — Unfractionated heparin
  — Low-molecular-weight heparin (LMWH; enoxaparin sodium [Lovenox])
- ACE inhibitors
  — Captopril (Capoten)
  — Enalapril sodium (Vasotec)
  — Benazepril hydrochloride (Lotensin)
- Analgesics
  — Morphine sulfate
- Discontinue any NSAID use.

Cholesterol-Lowering Drugs

These drugs may be initiated if dietary modification is unsuccessful.

- Atorvastatin calcium (Lipitor)
- Simvastatin (Zocor)
- Nicotinic acid (Niacin)

Oxygen

- Administer at 4 to 6 L/min to assist in oxygenating myocardial tissue in those hypoxic, in respiratory distress, or at high risk.

Nitroglycerin

- Dilates the coronary arteries.
- Increases blood flow to the damaged area of myocardium.
- Dosage
  — 0.4 mg/tablet
  — 1 tab sublingual q 5 minutes × 3 doses

Morphine Sulfate

- Analgesic
- ↓ Anxiety and tachypnea
- Relaxes bronchial smooth muscle.
- Improves gas exchange.

Thrombolytic Therapy

- Useful when infarction is diagnosed early and administered within protocol guidelines. There is a time imperative.
- Streptokinase, alteplase, or tPA
  — Administered IV
  — Most effective if given within 6 hours of onset of chest pain
- Heparin therapy usually follows thrombolytic therapy.

β-Blockers

- Decrease the heart rate.
- Reduce the workload of the heart.
- Decrease the oxygen demand of myocardium.

Calcium Channel Blockers

- Decrease conduction through the AV node.
- Slow the heart rate.
- Decrease the oxygen demand by the myocardium.

Medical Interventions

- Percutaneous transluminal coronary angioplasty (PTCA)
  — Balloon angioplasty
- Intracoronary stents
- Coronary artery bypass graft (CABG) really bad

Acute Myocardial Infarction

- Destruction of myocardial tissue due to lack of blood and oxygen supply
- Begins with occlusion of the coronary artery.
- Ischemia, injury, and infarction

- ST-segment elevation myocardial infarction (STEMI)
- Non-STEMI

Ischemia
- Results from reduced blood flow and oxygen to the coronary arteries
- If not reversed, injury occurs.
- Ischemia lasting 20 minutes or longer is sufficient to produce irreversible tissue damage.
- ST depression on ECG

Injury
- Prolonged interruption of oxygen supply and nutrients
- Cells still salvageable
- ST depression on ECG

Infarction
- Tissue necrosis and death
- Irreversible damage
- Scar tissue has no electrical stimulation or contractility.
- Within 24 hours of infarction, healing process begins.
- Pathological Q waves

Complications
- As many as 90% of clients suffer complications including:
  — Dysrhythmias
  — Cardiac failure
  — Cardiogenic shock
  — Thromboembolism
  — Ventricular rupture

Signs and Symptoms
- Pain
  — Sudden onset; severity increases
  — May persist for hours or days; not relieved by rest or nitroglycerin.
  — Heavy/constrictive
  — Located behind the sternum
  — May radiate to arms, back, neck, or jaw.
- Cool, clammy skin
- Rapid, irregular, feeble pulse

Atypical Symptoms
- Women
  — Discomfort rather than pain
  — Shortness of breath
  — Extreme fatigue
- Clients with diabetes
  — Asymptomatic
  — Neuropathy
  — Dyspnea
- Elderly clients
  — Confusion/delirium
  — Change in mental status
  — Dizziness
  — Shortness of breath

Medical Diagnosis

- ECG (12 lead): ST-segment elevation, T-wave inversion, and pathologic Q-wave formation
- Confirm by cardiac biomarkers.
- CK-MB
- Myoglobin
- Troponin

Cardiac Lab Tests

- Troponin level
  - Troponins found only in cardiac muscle.
  - May present as early after injury.
  - Peaks within 24 hours.
  - Returns to normal in 5 to 14 days.
- Myoglobin level
  - Myoglobin released 1 hour after an acute myocardial infarction (MI).
  - Rises before creatine kinase–MB levels
  - Returns to normal within 24 hours

Nursing and Collaborative Management

- Overall goal: reperfuse and preserve myocardial tissue
- Drug therapy
  - Oxygen
  - Nitroglycerin
  - Beta-blockers
  - Morphine
  - Thrombolytic therapy if PCI is not available
    - Administer within 120 minutes.
    - Avoid if symptoms >12 hours
- Percutaneous coronary intervention (PCI) and stents
  - Standard of care is PCI within 90 minutes of presentation for medical care.
  - If PCI is unavailable, then risk versus benefit ratio for thrombolytic therapy is completed.
- Coronary artery bypass graft
  - Used for severe coronary artery disease.
- Can be emergent or elective procedure.

Heart Failure
Etiology

- CAD, prior MI
- Chronic HTN
- Cardiomyopathy: dilated
- Idiopathic
- Thyroid
- Diabetes
- Restrictive
- Ischemic
- Valvular and congenital heart disease
- Pulmonary diseases

Left-Sided Heart Failure (LHF) *usually first*

- Causes: LV infarct, cardiomyopathy, and chronic uncontrolled hypertension
- Symptoms: dyspnea, cough, and fluid accumulation in the lungs

- Signs: tachycardia, inspiratory rales beginning at lung bases, and expiratory wheezes due to bronchospasms (misdiagnosed with asthma)
- Laboratory findings: ABGs reveal hypoxemia; chest x-ray study shows pulmonary edema or pleural effusions; B-type natriuretc peptide (BNP) levels >500 ng/mL indicate Heart Failure (HF) very probable

Right-Sided Heart Failure (RHF) Systemic Congestion

tries to take over
blood backs up into body

- Causes: LHF, RV infarct, pulmonary or tricuspid valve disease, pulmonary HTN, COPD, and PE
- Symptoms: dyspnea on exertion, fatigue, weight gain, and fluid retention
- Signs: increased central venous pressure (CVP), jugular venous distention (JVD), hepatomegaly, ascites, peripheral or sacral edema; pleural and pericardial effusions are also common.

Sodium and Volume Homeostasis

- As CO decreases, renal perfusion decreases.
- This activates the renin-angiotensin system and causes fluid retention.

Pharmacological Management

- Angiotensin-converting enzyme (ACE) inhibitors
  — Captopril
  — Enalapril sodium
  — Lisinopril
- Diuretics
  — Loop diuretics: furosemide
  — Thiazides: hydrochlorothiazide
  — Aldosterone antagonists: spironolactone
- Inotropes
  — Digoxin
  — Dobutamine hydrochloride
- Phosphodiesterase inhibitors
  — Milrinone
- Natriuretic peptides
  — Nesiritide
- β-blockers
  — Metoprolol
  — Carvedilol
  — Bisoprolol
- Angiotensin II receptor blockers
  — Losartan potassium
  — Candesartan cilexetil
  — Valsartan
- Vasodilators
  — Nitrates: isosorbide dinitrate
  — Hydralazine hydrochloride
  — Sodium nitroprusside
  — Prazosin hydrochloride
- Dopamine agonist
  — Dopamine hydrochloride
- Analgesics
  — Morphine sulfate
- Anticoagulants
  — Warfarin

- Antiplatelet
  - Aspirin
  - Clopidogrel
  - Ticlopidine

Nursing and Collaborative Management

- Reposition and perform coughing and deep breathing exercises every 2 hours.
- Diet
  - Limit sodium intake.
  - Restrict fluids only if $Na^+ < 132$ mg/dL.
  - Avoid excessive fluids.
  - Avoid alcohol, which depresses myocardial contractility.
  - With CAD: low cholesterol, low fat, and low Na^+
- Educate client on signs of worsening condition such as weight gain, increasing dyspnea on exertion, orthopnea, or paroxysmal nocturnal dyspnea.

The PN is administering 0900 medications to three clients on a telemetry unit when the unlicensed assistive personnel (UAP) reports that another client is complaining of a sudden onset of substernal discomfort. What action should the PN take?
A. Ask the UAP to obtain the client's vital signs.
B. Assess the client's discomfort.
C. Advise the client to rest in bed.
D. Observe the client's ECG pattern.

HESI Test Question Approach			
Positive?		**YES**	**NO**
Key Words			
Rephrase			
Rule Out Choices			
A	B	C	D

A client complains of a severe headache after receiving nitroglycerin 0.4 mg SL for angina. What prescription should the PN administer?
A. A second dose of nitroglycerin
B. A scheduled dose of low-dose aspirin
C. A PRN dose of acetaminophen PO
D. A PRN dose of morphine sulfate IM

HESI Test Question Approach			
Positive?		**YES**	**NO**
Key Words			
Rephrase			
Rule Out Choices			
A	B	C	D

Dysrhythmias: Interpretation and Management

- Standard ECG using 12 leads
  - Provides best overall evaluation
- Telemetry usually uses three leads that show one view of the heart.

- Holter monitor is usually worn for 24 hours to provide a continuous reading.

Electrocardiogram (ECG)
- P wave
  - Atrial depolarization
- QRS complex
  - Ventricular depolarization
  - Normal: <0.11 second
- ST segment
  - Early ventricular repolarization
- PR interval
  - Time for impulse to travel through SA node
  - Normal: 0.12 to 0.20 second
- R-R interval
  - Measures regularity of the heartbeat.

Dysrhythmias
- Client may be asymptomatic until cardiac output is altered.
- Client may complain of palpitations, syncope, pain, dyspnea, and diaphoresis.
- Changes occur in pulse rate/rhythm and ECG.
- Always treat the client and not the monitor!

Atrial Dysrhythmias
- A-fib (atrial fibrillation)
  - Chaotic activity in the AV node
  - No true P waves visible
  - Irregular ventricular rhythm
  - Risk for CVA
  - Anticoagulant therapy is necessary.
- Atrial flutter
  - Sawtoothed waveform
  - Fluttering in chest
  - Ventricular rhythm regular
    - Cardioversion may be used to treat either atrial dysrhythmia.

Ventricular Dysrhythmias
- V-tach (ventricular tachycardia)
  - Wide, bizarre QRS complex
  - Assess whether client has a pulse.
  - Prepare for synchronized cardioversion.
  - Administer antiarrhythmic drugs.
- V-fib (ventricular fibrillation)
  - Cardiac emergency
  - No cardiac output
  - Start cardiopulmonary resuscitation (CPR) per AHA guidelines.
  - Defibrillate as quickly as possible.
  - Administer antiarrhythmic drugs.

Antiarrhythmic Medications
- Class I: Sodium channel blockers reduce conduction velocity in the atria, ventricles, and His-Purkinje system.
  - IA
    - Disopyramide (Norpace)
    - Procainamide (Pronestyl)
    - Quinidine

—IB
- Lidocaine (Xylocaine)
- Mexiletine (Mexitil)
- Phenytoin (Dilantin)
- Tocainide (Tonocard)

—IC
- Flecainide (Tambocor)
- Propafenone (Rythmol)

- Class II: β-adrenergic blockers reduce automaticity of the SA node and decrease conduction velocity in the AV node.
  — Atenolol (Tenormin)
  — Metoprolol (Lopressor)
  — Sotalol (Betapace)
- Class III: Potassium channel blockers delay repolarization.
  — Amiodarone (Cordarone)
  — Dofetilide (Tikosyn)
- Class IV: Calcium channel blockers reduce automaticity of the SA node and delay AV node conduction.
  — Diltiazem (Cardizem)
  — Verapamil (Calan)
- Other antidysrhythmic drugs
  — Adenosine (Adenocard)
  — Digoxin (Lanoxin)
  — Magnesium

Inflammatory Heart Disease

Endocarditis

- S/S: fever, positive blood cultures, murmur, Osler nodes, Janeway's lesions, splinter hemorrhages, and heart failure symptoms; seen often with IV drug abuse.
- Infective endocarditis can lead to damaged heart valves.
- Assess for right- or left-sided heart failure.
- Administer IV antibiotics; therapy will continue for 4 to 6 weeks.
- Maintain balance of rest.
- Surgical treatment if valvular damage occurs
- Teach clients to request prophylactic antibiotics for every invasive procedure (dental included).

Pericarditis

- S/S: The pain hurts more when supine, with deep breathing or deep inhalations, pericardial friction rub.
- Facilitate a leaning-over position and NSAIDs for pain control measures.

Valvular Heart Disease

- Valves may be unable to
  — Fully open (stenosis)
  — Fully close (insufficiency or regurgitation)

Causes

- Rheumatic fever
- Congenital heart disease
- Syphilis

anything foreign will attract clots

- Endocarditis
- Hypertension

Mitral Valve Stenosis

- Early period: May be asymptomatic.
- Later period: excessive fatigue, dyspnea on exertion, orthopnea, dry cough, hemoptysis, or pulmonary edema — Murmur and a-fib are common.

Nursing and Collaborative Management

- See section on heart failure.
- Monitor for a-fib with thrombus formation.
- Encourage prophylactic antibiotic therapy before any invasive procedures (dental, surgical, or childbirth).
- Surgical repair or valve replacement may be required.
- With artificial valve replacement: Teach the client about the need for lifelong anticoagulant therapy.

Vascular Disorders

Arterial

- Smooth, shiny skin
- Pallor on elevation
- Weak or absent peripheral pulses
- Sharp or tingling pain
- Cool to touch
- Intermittent claudication (classic symptom)
- Painful, nonedematous ulcers

Venous

- Monitor for history of deep vein thrombosis.
- Bluish-purple skin discoloration
- Normal peripheral pulses
- Warm to touch
- Slightly painful ulcers with marked edema

Nursing and Collaborative Management

General

- Change positions frequently; avoid sitting with crossed legs.
- Do not wear restrictive clothing.
- Keep extremities warm with clothing and not external heaters.
- Discourage smoking.
- With thrombosis: Administer thrombolytic agents.

Arterial

- Bed rest
- Keep extremity below the level of the heart.
- Topical antibiotics
- Antiplatelet
- Surgical grafting intervention

Venous

- Wound care
- Diet that promotes wound healing includes zinc and vitamins A and C
- Compression stockings day and evening
- Elevate legs for at least 20 minutes, four to five times per day.

artey - feel cold
cap refill slow

venous - surface
- injury
warm skin

Abdominal Aortic Aneurysm

- Pulsating abdominal mass
- Bruit heard over abdomen
- Confirmed on x-ray study
- Rupture produces S/S of hypovolemic shock.
- Postoperative care for surgical repair
- Monitor for S/S of renal failure, postoperative ileus.
- Changes in pulses, S/S of occluded graft

Thrombophlebitis

- Inflammation of the venous wall with clot formation
- S/S: calf pain, edema of calf, induration (hardening) along the blood vessel, warmth and redness

NOTE: Pain in the calf on dorsiflexion of the foot (+ Homan's sign) appears in only a small percentage of clients with DVT, and false-positive findings are common. Therefore, relying on a Homan's sign is not advised.

- Restrict ambulation.
- Elevate extremity.
- Antiembolic stockings
- Refrain from massaging leg muscles.
- Medications
  — Heparin therapy
    - Therapeutic levels of aPTTs are usually 1½ to 2 times normal control levels.
    - Protamine sulfate antidote
  — Coumadin therapy
    - Monitor prothrombin time (PT), international normalized ratio (INR).
    - Vitamin K: antidote
  — Antiplatelet agents
    - Ticlopidine (Ticlid)
    - Clopidogrel bisulfate (Plavix)

The charge nurse assigns the PN clients on the acute care unit. Which client should the PN assess first?

A. A client receiving oxygen per nasal cannula who is dyspneic with mild exertion and has a hemoglobin of 7 g/dL

B. A client receiving IV aminoglycosides per CVC who complains of nausea and has a trough level below therapeutic levels

C. The client with heart failure with sudden onset of shortness of breath and a BNP level of 800 pg/mL

D. A client receiving chemotherapy who has a temperature of 98.9°F and a WBC count of 2500/mm^3

HESI Test Question Approach		
Positive?	YES	NO
Key Words		
Rephrase		
Rule Out Choices		
A	B	C	D

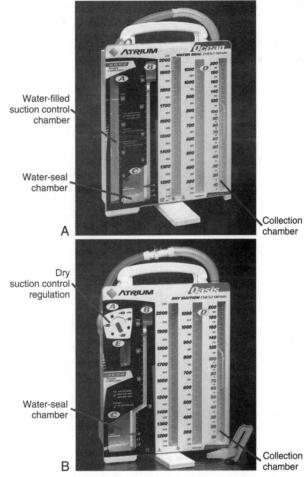

Water-filled suction control chamber

Water-seal chamber

Collection chamber

A

Dry suction control regulation

Water-seal chamber

Collection chamber

B

Fig. 5-1 Chest tubes are used to remove or drain blood or air from the intrapleural space, to expand the lung after surgery, or to restore subatmospheric pressure to the thoracic cavity. Many brands of commercial chest drainage systems are available; all are based on the traditional three-bottle, water seal system. Picture (A) is a commonly used disposable chest drainage system and (B) is a diagram of the chambers of a water seal chest drainage system. (Lewis, S., Dirksen, S., Heitkemper, M., Bucher, L. (2014). *Medical-surgical nursing: Assessment and management of clinical problems* (9th ed.). St. Louis, MO, Mosby, Fig. 28-8, p. 545.)

6 Ingestion, Digestion, Absorption, and Elimination

While obtaining the health history of a client and reviewing his medical records, which data will alert the PN that the client has an increased risk of developing peptic ulcer disease? (Select all that apply.)

A. Excess of gastric acid or a decrease in the natural ability of the GI mucosa to protect itself from acid and pepsin
B. Invasion of the stomach and/or duodenum by *H. pylori*
C. Viral infection, allergies to certain foods, immunologic factors, and psychosomatic factors
D. Taking certain drugs, including corticosteroids and antiinflammatory medications
E. Having allergies to foods that contain gluten

HESI Test Question Approach			
Positive?		YES	NO
Key Words			
Rephrase			
Rule Out Choices			
A	B	C	D	E

Gastroesophageal Reflux Disease (GERD)

- Any clinically significant symptomatic condition secondary to reflux of gastric contents into the lower esophagus
- The most common upper GI problem seen in adults but can occur in all age groups
- There is no single cause of GERD.
- Predisposing conditions include:
  — Incompetent lower esophageal sphincter (LES)
  — Hiatal hernia
  — Decreased esophageal clearance (ability to clear liquids or food from the esophagus into the stomach)
  — Decreased gastric emptying

Nursing Assessment

- Heartburn after eating
- Eructation
- Fullness and discomfort after eating
- Diagnostics
  — Esophageal pH and mobility testing (LES, GI, and esophageal motility issues); barium swallow with fluoroscopy hiatal hernia); endoscopy

Nursing and Collaborative Management

- Treatment options: symptom management and options directed toward the predisposing issue
- Medications
  — Antacids neutralize or reduce acidity of stomach contents (Maalox, Gaviscon, Rolaids, Tums, Mylanta, and Riopan)
  — H$_2$ receptor antagonists decrease acid secretions by blocking histamine receptors; can increase effects and serum levels of oral anticoagulants, theophylline, phenytoin, some benzodiazepines, and

propranolol (Cimetidine [Tagamet], ranitidine [Zantac], famotidine [Pepcid], or nizatidine [Axid]).
— Proton pump inhibitors (PPIs) inhibit gastrin secretion—Omeprazole (Prilosec) inhibits hepatic metabolism of warfarin, phenytoin, benzodiazepines, and other drugs metabolized by liver. Do not crush or chew capsule contents of esomeprazole (Nexium), pantoprazole (Protonix), rabeprazole (AcipHex), and lansoprazole (Prevacid).
— Mucosal healing agent (Sucralfate [Carafate])
— Promotility agents (Metoclopramide [Reglan])
- Procedures to consider to strengthen LES:
— Nissen fundoplication, Stretta procedure
— Monitor for Barrett's esophagus
- Lifestyle modifications
— Avoid foods and beverages that cause heartburn
— Smoking cessation
— Weight management
— Encourage small, frequent meals.
— Sit up while eating and remain upright for 1 hour after eating.
— Stop eating 3 hours before bedtime.
— Elevate head of bed 4 to 6 inches.

Peptic Ulcer Disease
- Ulcerations of the mucous membrane or other layers of the GI tract, most commonly occurring in the stomach and duodenum. Most common between the ages of 55 and 65 years.
- Most common causes include *H. pylori* bacteria, regular use of NSAIDs, smoking or chewing tobacco, excessive alcohol, and stress.

Nursing Assessment
- Left epigastric pain that may radiate to back; can also include nausea, weight loss, eructation, and distention.
- Symptoms occur 1 to 2 hours after meals and intensify with perforation or obstruction.
- Epigastric pain is usually relieved with food.
- Diagnostic procedures
— Esophagogastroduodenoscopy (EGD), Barium swallow, and testing for *H. pylori*

Nursing and Collaborative Management
Medication management to control symptoms and reduce acid includes antacids, H2 receptor blockers, Proton pump inhibitors, mucosal healing agents, and cytoprotective agents (misoprostol [Cytotec]).

Antibiotics to eradicate *H. pylori* include metronidazole (Flagyl), tetracycline, amoxicillin, clarithromycin (Biaxin), and Helidac (14-day supply of bismuth, metronidazole, and tetracycline to increase compliance).

Surgery may be needed for complications (i.e., perforation, hemorrhage, penetration, or gastric outlet obstruction).

Complications
- Dumping syndrome (rapid gastric emptying of undigested food from the stomach to the small intestine causing distention of the duodenum or jejunum) occurs in one-third to one-half of clients following surgery for peptic ulcers.

— Symptoms include nausea, vomiting, diaphoresis, explosive diarrhea, and changes in blood glucose levels.

— Management includes eating six small meals daily that are high in protein and fat and low in carbohydrates, eating slowly, avoiding fluids during meals, giving anticholinergic agents to decrease stomach motility, and reclining for approximately 1 hour after meals. Reassure client that symptoms will decrease and disappear within a year after surgery.

Client Teaching

- Lifestyle modifications include eating small, frequent meals; smoking cessation; and avoiding foods that irritate the GI mucosa.
- History of symptoms (precipitating and alleviating factors)
- Instruct client to monitor for hematemesis and melena.

Crohn's Disease (Regional Enteritis)

Chronic disorder characterized by inflammation of segments of the GI tract.

- The cause is unknown, but possibly includes autoimmune, genetic, and environmental factors.
- Onset is early adolescence; second peak is in sixth decade
- Occurs anywhere along the GI tract (most common site is terminal ileum and proximal cecum).
- Inflammation can be continuous or intermittent and extends through all layers of intestine. Areas impacted have a cobblestone appearance.
- Clients are likely to develop bowel obstruction, fistulas, fissures, and abscesses. Surgical interventions are most often needed for these secondary complications.

Nursing Assessment

- Right lower quadrant abdominal pain, nausea, vomiting, weight loss, fever, dehydration steatorrhea (three to four stools per day, no blood present in stool), and unexplained anemia
- Barium enema with small bowel follow-through

Nursing and Collaborative Management

Goal is to achieve remission with first-line drugs.

- Antiinflammatory agents (sulfasalazine, mesalamine, olsalazine, or balsalazide)
- Multivitamins and B_{12} injections
- During severe inflammation client will be NPO, and TPN will be used to allow bowel rest.
- Monitor weight.
- Encourage at least 2–3 L of fluid per day
- Instruct client in low-residue, high-protein, high-calorie diet (limited dairy).
- Emotional support
- Support group referral: Crohn's and Colitis Foundation of America (http://www.crohnscolitisfoundation.org/)

Ulcerative Colitis

Ulcerative colitis is confined to the mucosa and submucosa of the colon.

- Cause is unknown but thought to be autoimmune or immune response and/or genetic predisposition.
- Complications seen less in ulcerative colitis include bleeding, rupture, and abdominal bloating. Toxic megacolon is rare but does occur.
- Surgical interventions include colon resection, ileostomy, proctocolectomy, and Kock pouch.

Nursing Assessment

- Bloody diarrhea, liquid stools: Severe is 10 to 20 per day and electrolyte imbalances.
- Fever, tachycardia, weight loss, abdominal cramping and pain, and anemia

Nursing and Collaborative Management

Conservative medical management with medications includes antiinflammatory agents (sulfasalazine [Azulfidine], olsalazine [Dipentum], mesalamine [Pentasa], and balsalazide [Colazal]), corticosteroids, antidiarrheal agents, diet, and stress reduction.

- Encourage elemental diet high in calories and lactose free.
- Tepid fluids
- Monitor weight and daily calorie count.
- Monitor intake and output (I & O)
- Emotional support

Diverticular Diseases

Diverticulosis is the presence of pouch-like herniations through the smooth muscle of the colon.

Diverticulitis is the inflammation of one or more of the diverticular sacs. Inflammation can lead to perforation, abscess, peritonitis, obstruction, and hemorrhage.

Associated risk factors are age > 40, lack of exercise, obesity, and smoking.

Nursing Assessment

- Left lower quadrant pain, fever, elevated WBC, and ESR
- Monitor for signs and symptoms of intestinal obstruction (abdominal distention, constipation and/or diarrhea).
- Ultrasound, CT scan, and colonoscopy

Nursing and Collaborative Management

- High-fiber diet (avoid foods containing seeds) unless inflammation is present
  — If inflammation is present:
- NPO
- Then low-residue, bland diet
- Bulk-forming laxatives
- Avoid heavy lifting, tight clothing, and straining.

Intestinal Obstruction

- Mechanical causes
  — Adhesions most common
  — Strangulated hernia
  — Tumors

- Neurogenic causes
  — Paralytic ileus
  — Spinal cord lesion
- Vascular cause
  — Mesenteric artery occlusion

Nursing Assessment
- Sudden abdominal pain
- History of obstruction
- High-pitched bowel sounds (early mechanical obstruction)
- Bowel sounds diminished or absent (neurogenic or late mechanical obstruction)

Nursing and Collaborative Management
- NPO
- Intravenous (IV) fluids
- Nasogastric tube to intermittent suction

Cirrhosis
Cirrhosis is a chronic, progressive disease in which the lobes of the liver become covered with scar tissue; the liver degenerates, and the lobules are infiltrated with fat.
- There are several forms of cirrhosis related to the associated cause (alcohol-related liver disease, postnecrotic cirrhosis, primary biliary cirrhosis, and cardiac cirrhosis).

Nursing Assessment
- Early sign: right upper quadrant pain
- Jaundice: yellow sclera
- Dark-colored urine
- Clay-colored stools
- Fruity or musty breath
- Asterixis
- Palmar erythema
- Ascites
- Weight loss
- Mental confusion
- Pruritis (bile salts)
- Lab findings: ↑serum bilirubin, AST, ALT, LDH, and GTT; ↓total protein and serum albumin; ↑ammonia; ↓blood glucose (hypoglycemia) from impaired gluconeogenesis; prolonged prothrombin time; ↑ INR; and ↓cholesterol levels
- An endoscopic retrograde cholangiopancreatography (ERCP) to detect common bile duct obstruction, esophagoscopy with barium esophagography to visualize esophageal varices, scans, a biopsy of the liver, and ultrasonography are used to diagnose cirrhosis.

Management of Esophageal Varices
- A common complication of cirrhosis associated with portal hypertension; may rupture and cause hemorrhage.
- A preventative to reduce the likelihood of rupture (propranolol [Inderal]) is used.
- If rupture occurs, this is a medical emergency.

Nursing and Collaborative Management

- Interventions to manage hemorrhage
  - Hemodynamic stability: fresh, frozen plasma and packed RBCs; vitamin K (AquaMEPHYTON); histamine (H2) receptor blockers such as cimetidine (Tagamet); and electrolyte replacements
  - Vasopressin (VP) administered intravenously or directly into the superior vena cava is used to decrease or stop the hemorrhaging (sometimes used concurrently with nitroglycerin).
  - Balloon tamponade (i.e., Sengstaken-Blakemore tube)
  - Octreotide (Sandostatin) is sometimes used in combination with band ligation.
- Treatment options to manage cirrhosis
  - Diuretics
  - Vitamin supplements include vitamin K, vitamin C, and folic acid
  - Lactulose (Chronulac) as ammonia detoxicant
- Instruct client regarding a well-balanced, moderate, high-protein (except in hepatic encephalopathy, then limit protein), high-carbohydrate diet with adequate vitamins.
- Monitor for bleeding, and instruct in bleeding precautions (Avoid injections, maintain pressure for 5 minutes after venipunctures, and use electric razor.).
- Provide skin care; avoid soap, perfumed lotions and rubbing alcohol; use mild lotions; diphenhydramine (Benadryl) may be used for pruritus.
- Monitor fluid, electrolytes, and ascites; determine accurate I & O; weigh daily; restrict fluids (1500 mL/day); measure abdominal girth; and plan for possible paracentesis and peritoneovenous (LeVeen continuous peritoneal jugular shunt).

Hepatitis

Widespread inflammation of liver cells, usually caused by a virus

- Hepatitis A (formerly called infectious hepatitis) is the most common form today and is a short-incubation virus (10 to 40 days).
- Hepatitis B (formerly called serum hepatitis) has a long incubation period (28 to 160 days).
- Hepatitis C has an incubation period of 2 weeks to 6 months (commonly 6 to 9 weeks).
- Hepatitis D (also called delta virus) causes hepatitis as a coinfection with hepatitis B and may progress to cirrhosis and chronic hepatitis. The incubation period is 2 to 10 weeks.
- Hepatitis E (also called enteric non-A–non-B hepatitis) is transmitted through fecal contamination of water, primarily in developing countries. It is rare in the United States. The incubation period is 15 to 64 days.
- Hepatitis G virus has been found in blood donors and can be transmitted by transfusion. It frequently coexists with other hepatitis viruses, such as hepatitis C.

If it ends in a vowel, it comes from the bowel.

Nursing Assessment

- Risk groups
  - Men who have sex with men
  - IV drug users (Disease is transmitted by contaminated needles.)
  - Tattooing or body piercing with contaminated needles
  - Persons living in crowded conditions
  - Healthcare workers employed in high-risk areas
- Fatigue, weakness
- Anorexia, nausea
- Jaundice
- Dark urine
- Joint pain, muscle aches
- Laboratory values
  - Increased direct bilirubin, GGT, AST, ALT, LDH, and alkaline phosphatase levels; a prolonged prothrombin time and ↑INR; in severe hepatitis, ↓serum albumin
  - Leukopenia (low white blood cell count) followed by lymphocytosis (high lymphocyte count)
  - Hypoglycemia is present in approximately 50% of patients with hepatitis.
  - Serum is examined for the presence of antigens associated with hepatitis A, B, C, D, or G.
  - A CT scan of the abdomen reveals hepatomegaly.

Nursing and Collaborative Management

- Frequent rest periods
- Provide high-calorie, high-carbohydrate diet with moderate fats and proteins.
- Administer antiemetic as needed.
- Limit alcohol intake and drugs detoxified by the liver.

Pancreatitis

- Acute: autodigestion of the pancreas
  - Alcohol ingestion and biliary tract disease
- Chronic: progressive, destructive disease
  - Long-term alcohol use

Acute Pancreatitis Assessment

Abdominal pain is the predominant symptom of acute pancreatitis.

- Located in the left upper quadrant
- Radiates to the back
- Sudden onset
- Described as severe, deep, piercing, and continuous
- Aggravated by eating and not relieved by vomiting
- Accompanied by flushing, cyanosis, and dyspnea

Other Manifestations of Acute Pancreatitis

- Nausea and vomiting
- Low-grade fever
- Jaundice
- Bowel sounds may be decreased or absent; ileus may occur.
- Hypotension
- Tachycardia
- Hypovolemia (massive fluid shift into the retroperitoneal space)

- Shock (hemorrhage into the pancreas)
- Crackles

Chronic Pancreatitis Assessment

- Steatorrhea
- Diarrhea
- Jaundice
- Ascites
- Weight loss

Nursing and Collaborative Management

- Acute management
  — NPO
  — NG tube to suction
  — Antispasmodic agents (Pro-Banthine)
  — Morphine for pain management
  — Sitting up or leaning forward may reduce pain.
  — Monitor blood sugar.
  — Teach foods and fluids to avoid.
- Chronic management
  — Pancreatic enzymes
- Creon
- Viokase
- Mix powdered forms with fruit juice or applesauce; avoid mixing with proteins.
  — Teach foods and fluids to avoid.
  — Support efforts to abstain from alcohol.
  — Antispasmodics

A client with an obstruction of the common bile duct caused by cholelithiasis passes clay-colored stools containing streaks of fat. What action should the practical nurse take?
A. Auscultate for diminished bowel sounds.
B. Send a stool specimen to the laboratory.
C. Document the assessment in the chart.
D. Notify the healthcare provider.

HESI Test Question Approach			
Positive?		YES	NO
Key Words			
Rephrase			
Rule Out Choices			
A	B	C	D

Cholecystitis and Cholelithiasis

- Cholecystitis (acute inflammation of the gallbladder) *CVRN*
- Cholelithiasis (formation or presence of gallstones) *surgery*

Nursing Assessment

- Pain
- Fever
- Elevated WBC count
- Abdominal tenderness
- Jaundice

Nursing and Collaborative Management

- Analgesics for pain
- NPO
- NG to suction

- IV antibiotics
- Low-fat diet (Avoid fried, spicy, and fatty foods.)

Cholelithiasis
- Nonsurgical removal
  —Endoscopic retrograde cholangiopancreatography (ERCP)
  —Lithotripsy
- Surgical approach
  —Cholecystectomy, laparoscopic or open

A client is admitted with gastric ulcer disease and GI bleeding. Which risk factor should the practical nurse identify in the client's history?
A. Eats heavily seasoned foods
B. Uses NSAIDs daily
C. Consumes alcohol every day
D. Follows an acid-ash diet

HESI Test Question Approach			
Positive?		YES	NO
Key Words			
Rephrase			
Rule Out Choices			
A	B	C	D

Renal and Urologic Problems

Urinary Tract Infections
- Obtain clean-catch midstream specimen.
- Administer antibiotics as ordered.
  —Complete prescribed dose.
  —Do not skip doses.
- Encourage fluid intake of 3000 mL/day.
- Encourage voiding every 2 to 3 hours.
- Avoid tight clothing and bubble baths.

Urinary Tract Obstruction
- Caused by calculi or stones
- Location of pain can help locate stone.
  —Flank pain (stone usually in upper ureter)
  —Pain radiating to abdomen (stone likely in ureter or bladder)

Nursing and Collaborative Management
- Administer narcotics.
- Strain all urine for passing stones. Encourage high fluid intake (3 to 4 L per day).
- Strict I & O
- Surgical management may be required.

Benign Prostatic Hyperplasia
Enlargement of the prostate
- Increased urinary frequency and decreased output
- Bladder distention (increases risk of spasm)
- Nonsurgical options for management:
  —Alpha-blockers (terazosin [Hytrin], doxazosin [Cardura], and tamsulosin [Flomax])

high volume fluid 24/hr
call MD if blood after 24 h

— 5-alpha-reductase inhibitors-finasteride (Proscar) and dutasteride (Avodart)
- Surgical options:
  — Transurethral microwave thermotherapy
  — Transurethral needle ablation (TUNA)
  — Photoselective vaporization of the prostate
  — Most common treatment is transurethral resection of the prostate (TURP).
  — If prostate is too large, use suprapubic approach.

Nursing and Collaborative Management
- Preoperative teaching
  — Pain management
  — Oversized balloon catheter
- Bladder spasms
  — Common after surgery
  — Use antispasmodics
  — Belladonna and opium suppositories
  — Oxybutynin chloride (Ditropan)
  — Dicyclomine hydrochloride (Bentylol)
- Continuous bladder irrigation is typically done to remove blood clots and ensure drainage.
- Drainage should be reddish pink for 24 hours, clearing to light pink.
- Monitor color and amount of urine output.
- Notify physician if client has bright red bleeding with large clots.

Discharge Teaching
- Continue to drink 12 to 14 glasses of water per day.
- Avoid straining.
- Avoid strenuous activity, sports, lifting, and intercourse for 3 to 4 weeks.
- Report large amounts of blood or frank blood.

A client is in the oliguric phase of acute kidney injury. Which of the following findings would the nurse expect to assess on the client? (Select all that apply.)
A. 450 mL urine output in 24 hours
B. Potassium of 6.2 mEq/L
C. Sodium (serum) 155 mEq/L
D. Metabolic alkalosis
E. Weight gain

HESI Test Question Approach			
Positive?		**YES**	**NO**
Key Words			
Rephrase			
Rule Out Choices			

A	B	C	D	E

A client who has acute renal failure is admitted to the hospital. The client's potassium level is 6.4 mEq/L. Which snack should the practical nurse offer?
A. An orange
B. A milkshake
C. Dried fruit and nuts
D. A gelatin dessert

HESI Test Question Approach			
Positive?		YES	NO
Key Words			
Rephrase			
Rule Out Choices			
A	B	C	D

Acute Kidney Injury
- It is a reversible syndrome if symptoms are caught early enough!
- Remember:
  — Kidneys use 25% of normal cardiac output to maintain function.
  — Kidneys excrete 1 to 2 L of urine per 24 hours for adults.
  — Three types of acute kidney injuries
    • Prerenal
    • Intrarenal
    • Postrenal

Prerenal Failure
- Etiologic factors
  — Hemorrhage
  — Hypovolemia
  — Decreased cardiac output
  — Decreased renal perfusion

Intrarenal Failure
- Etiologic factors
  — May develop secondary to prerenal failure
  — Nephrotoxins
  — Infections (glomerulonephritis)
  — Renal injury
  — Vascular lesions

Postrenal Failure
- Etiologic factors for obstruction
  — Calculi
  — Benign prostatic hyperplasia (BPH)
  — Tumors
  — Strictures

Nursing Assessment
- Decreased urine output
- Weight gain
- Edema
- Diagnostic test results: oliguric phase

— ↓ Urine output
— ↑ Blood urea nitrogen (BUN) and creatinine
— ↑ Potassium
— ↓ Sodium (serum)
— ↓ pH
— Metabolic acidosis
— ↑ Urine sodium
— Fixed at 1.010, specific gravity
■ Diagnostic test results: diuretic phase
— ↑ Urine output
— ↓ Fluid volume
— ↓ Potassium
— ↓ Sodium
— ↓ Urine specific gravity
— ↓ Urine sodium

Nursing and Collaborative Management
■ In oliguric phase, give only enough fluids to replace losses > 400 to 500 mL/24 hr.
■ Strict I & O
■ Monitor laboratory values closely.
■ Watch for ECG changes.
■ Monitor weight daily.

The nurse is evaluating blood results for a client with end-stage renal disease who has just undergone hemodialysis. Which value should the nurse verify with the laboratory?
A. Elevated serum potassium
B. Increase in serum calcium
C. Low hemoglobin
D. Reduction in serum sodium

HESI Test Question Approach		
Positive?	**YES**	**NO**
Key Words		
Rephrase		
Rule Out Choices		
A	B	C	D

Chronic Kidney Disease (CKD)
■ End-stage renal disease
■ Progressive, irreversible damage to the nephrons and glomeruli
■ Causes
— Diabetic nephropathy
— Hypertensive nephrosclerosis
— Glomerulonephritis
— Polycystic kidney disease

Nursing Assessment
■ Early stage
— Polyuria
— Renal insufficiency
■ Late stage
— Oliguria
— Hematuria
— Proteinuria
— Edema
— Increased BP

—Muscle wasting, secondary to negative nitrogen balance

—Ammonia taste in mouth

—↑ Creatinine, ↑ phosphorus, ↑ potassium

■ End stage

—Anuria (<100 mL/24 hr)

Nursing and Collaborative Management

■ Monitor serum electrolytes.

■ Weigh daily.

■ Strict I & O

■ Renal diet

—Low protein

—Low sodium

—Low potassium

—Low phosphate

Medications

■ Drugs to manage associated complications

—Aluminum hydroxide (to bind phosphates)

—Epoetin to treat anemia (Epogen)

—Antihypertensive therapy

—Calcium supplements and vitamin D

—Antihyperlipidemics

—Statins to lower LDL

—Fibrates to lower triglycerides

CAUTION: As kidney function decreases, medication dosages must be adjusted.

Renal Dialysis

■ Hemodialysis

—AV fistula

■ No venipunctures, IVs, or BP in AV shunt arm

■ Withhold medications that would affect hemodynamic stability before dialysis.

■ Peritoneal dialysis

—Monitor indwell and outflow times closely.

—Monitor I & O.

Postoperative Care: Kidney Surgery

■ Respiratory status

—Auscultate to detect wet sounds.

—Demonstrate splinting method.

■ Circulatory status

—Monitor for shock.

—Monitor surgical site for bleeding.

■ Pain relief status

—Administer narcotic analgesics as needed.

■ Urinary status

—Check urinary output and drainage from **all** tubes.

—Strict I & O

7 Regulatory, Reproductive, and Urinary

A client who has type 1 diabetes returns to the clinic for follow-up after dietary counseling. The client states that he has been managing his diabetes closely. Which laboratory result indicates the client is maintaining tight control of the disease?
A. FBS changes from (135 to 110 mg/dL)
B. SMBG at bedtime changes from 45 to 90 mg/dL
C. Glycosylated hemoglobin (hemoglobin A1c) changes from 9% to 6%
D. Urine ketones change from 0 to 3

HESI Test Question Approach		
Positive?	YES	NO
Key Words		
Rephrase		
Rule Out Choices		
A	B	C	D

Obesity, Metabolic Syndrome, Prediabetes, and Diabetes

Primary Obesity

Primary obesity results when a person's caloric intake exceeds the body's metabolic rate.
- Assessed using a body mass index (BMI) chart
  - Normal weight: BMI $= 18.5$ to 24.9 kg/m^2
  - Overweight: BMI $= 25$ to 29.9 kg/m^2
  - Obese: BMI ≥ 30 kg/m^2
  - Morbidly obese: BMI > 40 kg/m^2
- Abdominal and visceral fat linked to metabolic syndrome
- Disproportionately represented in minority populations

Nursing Assessment
- Risk factor screening
  - Cardiovascular disease
  - Hypertension
  - Sleep apnea
  - Type 2 diabetes

Nursing and Collaborative Management
- Lifestyle management
  - Medical and nutritional therapy
  - Physical activity
  - Behavior modification
- Pharmacological therapy
- Bariatric surgery
  - Criteria for bariatric surgery
    - BMI ≥ 40 kg/m^2 *or*
    - BMI ≥ 35 kg/m^2 with one or more medical complications related to severe obesity
  - Gastric bypass, gastric banding, and Roux-en-Y

Metabolic Syndrome

Metabolic syndrome is a collection of risk factors that increase an individual's chance of developing cardiovascular disease and diabetes mellitus.

Nursing Assessment

- The client meets three or more of the following criteria:
  — Waist circumference
    - Men: $\geq$40 inches (102 cm)
    - Women: $\geq$35 inches (88 cm)
  — Triglycerides >150 mg/dL or drug treatment for elevated triglycerides
  — High-density lipoprotein (HDL)
    - <40 mg/dL in men; <50 mg/dL in women
    - Drug treatment for reduced HDL cholesterol
  — Low-density lipoprotein (LDL)
    - <2.6 mmol/L (<100 mg/dL)
  — BP $\geq$ 130 mm Hg systolic or $\geq$85 mm Hg diastolic or drug treatment for hypertension
  — Fasting blood glucose level (100 mg/dL)

Nursing and Collaborative Management

- Lifestyle management

Prediabetes

Prediabetes is a condition in which individuals are at an increased risk of developing diabetes.

- Fasting blood glucose levels: 100 to 125 mg/dL
- 2-hour oral glucose tolerance test (OGTT): <140 mg/dL
- Hemoglobin A_{1C}: 5.7% to 6.4%

Diabetes Mellitus

Diabetes mellitus (DM) is a chronic, multisystem disease related to abnormal insulin production, impaired insulin utilization, or both.

- Type 1 diabetes is an immune-mediated disease: T cells attack and destroy beta cells, the source of insulin, causing absolute insulin deficiency.
- Type 2 diabetes mellitus: The basic defect is insulin resistance and relative insulin deficiency.

Clinical Manifestations

- Type 1
  — Rapid onset
  — Can occur at any age, but onset typically is seen in childhood or adolescence.
  — Classic symptoms: polyuria, polydipsia, polyphagia, and weight loss
  — Weakness and fatigue are also possible.
  — Ketoacidosis is possible.
- Type 2
  — Risk factors
    - Age > 45 years
    - BMI > 25 (overweight)
    - First-degree relative with diabetes
    - Sedentary lifestyle
    - At-risk ethnic group
    - History of gestational diabetes or baby >9 lb
    - Cardiovascular comorbidity

- Onset is insidious with polyuria, polyphagia, polydipsia, and weight loss; client may experience fatigue, recurrent infections, prolonged wound healing, blurred vision, impotence.
- Development of ketoacidosis (rare)
- Client with blood glucose level >600 mg/dL is likely to develop hyperosmolar hyperglycemia nonketotic syndrome (HHNKS).

■ Other types of diabetes
- Cystic fibrosis–related diabetes
- Transplant-related diabetes
- Gestational diabetes
- Steroid-induced diabetes
- Hospital-related hyperglycemia

Diagnostic Studies
Any of four tests can be used to diagnose type 1 or type 2 diabetes mellitus
- Glycosylated hemoglobin (HgbA$_{1C}$): $\geq$ 6.5%
- Fasting plasma glucose (FPG): 100 to 125 mg/dL
- 2-hour OGTT (75-g glucose load): <140 mg/dL
- Random blood glucose level >200 mg/dL accompanied by classic symptoms of hyperglycemia (polyuria, polydipsia, polyphagia, and unexplained weight loss)

Those in high-risk groups should have an annual screening.

Nursing Assessment
■ Integument: skin breakdown
■ Eyes: retinal problems, cataracts
■ Kidneys: edema, urinary retention
■ Periphery: cool skin
■ Ulcerations on extremities and thick nails
■ Cardiopulmonary angina and dyspnea

Nursing and Collaborative Management
■ Teach injection techniques.
■ Refrigerate unopened insulin.
■ Eat a heart-healthy diet with consistent carbohydrate intake, proteins 15%–20%, and saturated fats <7%.
■ Physical activity
■ Integrate meals and snacks, insulin therapy, and physical activity.
■ May need a snack before or during exercise.
■ Monitor for signs and symptoms of hypoglycemia.
■ Foot care
- Check feet daily
- Report signs of injury
■ Managing sick days
- Continue insulin.
- Check blood sugar more frequently.
- Watch for signs and symptoms of hyperglycemia.

The PN is assigned a client with diabetes. Which findings should the PN report immediately? (Select all that apply.)

A. Finger stick blood sugar 247 mg/dL
B. Cold, clammy skin
C. Crackles at end of inspiration
D. Numbness in fingertips and toes
E. Unsteady gait, slurred speech

HESI Test Question Approach			
Positive?		**YES**	**NO**
Key Words			
Rephrase			
Rule Out Choices			

A	B	C	D	E

Oral Antidiabetic Agents

Oral antidiabetic agents are not insulin. These drugs work on the three defects of type 2 diabetes: (1) insulin resistance, (2) decreased insulin production, and (3) increased hepatic glucose production.

Types of Oral Antidiabetic Drugs

- Sulfonylureas increase insulin production from the pancreas; therefore, hypoglycemia is a major side effect.
  - Glipizide
  - Glimepiride (Amaryl) (take with meal)
- Meglitinides increase insulin production from the pancreas; they are more rapidly absorbed and eliminated than sulfonylureas and therefore less likely to cause hypoglycemia. Take 15 minutes before a meal.
  - Repaglinide
  - Nateglinide
- Biguanides reduce glucose production by liver and enhance insulin sensitivity at tissue level; they are a first-choice drug for most people with type 2 diabetes. Do not use in clients with kidney disease, liver disease, heart failure, or in clients who drink excessive amounts of alcohol.
  - Metformin
- The α-glucosidase inhibitors (starch blockers) slow the absorption of carbohydrate in the small intestine.
  - Acarbose
- Thiazolidinediones (insulin sensitizers) are most effective for clients with insulin resistance and do not cause hypoglycemia when used alone. Do not use thiazolidinediones in clients with heart failure because of ↑risk of myocardial infarction and stroke.
  - Pioglitazone hydrochloride
  - Rosiglitazone maleate
- Dipeptidyl peptidase-4 (DPP-4) inhibitors inhibit DPP-4, slowing the inactivation of incretin hormones. Because DPP-4 inhibitors are glucose dependent, they lower the potential for hypoglycemia. May take DPP-4 s with or without food.
  - Sitagliptin

- Incretin mimetic simulates one of the incretin hormones found to decrease in people with type 2 diabetes. A prefilled pen is used to administer the drug subcutaneously. Acute pancreatitis and kidney problems have been associated with the use of these drugs.
    — Exenatide (Byetta)
- Amylin analog is a synthetic analog of human amylin; it is indicated for clients with type 1 diabetes and for those with type 2 diabetes who have not achieved glucose control despite the use of insulin at mealtimes. This drug is administered subcutaneously and cannot be mixed with insulin; severe hypoglycemia can result if the drug is used with insulin.

Insulin Pharmacokinetics after Subcutaneous Injection

Rapid-Acting Insulin Can Be Given IV
- Glulisine is given within 15 minutes of meal.
    — Onset: 15 minutes
    — Peak: 1 hour
    — Duration: 2 to 3 hours
- Lispro is given within 15 minutes of meal.
    — Onset: 15 minutes
    — Peak: 1 hour
    — Duration: 4 hours
- Aspart is given within 15 minutes of meal.
    — Onset: 30 minutes
    — Peak: 1 to 3 hours
    — Duration: 3 to 5 hours
- Regular insulin is given within 30 minutes of meal.
    — Onset: 30 minutes to 1 hour
    — Peak: 2 to 4 hours
    — Duration: 5 to 7 hours

Intermediate-Acting Insulin: Do not give IV; can be mixed with rapid-acting insulins (See Combinations section, below.)
- Insulin isophane suspension (Humulin N)
    — Onset: 1 to 2 hours
    — Peak: 4 to 8 hours
    — Duration: 10 to 18 hours

Long-Acting Insulin: Cannot be mixed with any other type of insulin. Usually it is given once a day in the morning. It acts as basal insulin. Do not shake solutions. CAUTION: Solution is clear. Do not confuse with regular insulin
- Glargine
    — Onset: 1 to 5 hours
    — Peak: Plateau
    — Duration: 24 hours
- Detemir
    — Onset: 3 to 4 hours
    — Peak: Peakless
    — Duration: 24 hours

Combinations (Premix Insulins)
- Regular insulin 30% and insulin isophane (Humulin N) 70%

— Onset: 30 minutes to 1 hour
— Peak: 1.5 to 12 hours
— Duration: up to 24 hours

- Lispro insulins: lispro protamine insulin suspension 75% and insulin lispro 25%
  — Onset: 15 to 30 min
  — Peak: ≥2 hours
  — Duration: about 22 hours
- Lispro insulins: lispro protamine suspension 50% and insulin lispro 50%
  — Onset: 15 to 30 min
  — Peak: 30 to 90 min
  — Duration: about 22 hours
- Aspart insulins: 30% soluble insulin aspart and 70% insulin aspart protamine crystals (NovoMix 30)
  — Onset: about 10 to 20 minutes
  — Peak: 1 to 4 hours
  — Duration: up to 24 hours

Because analog premixed insulin has a rapid onset, it should be given shortly before meals and should not be given at bedtime. Clients who choose to use premixed insulin preparations should have a fairly routine lifestyle.

In clients with impaired liver or kidney function, the insulin dosage may need to be reduced because insulin is metabolized by the liver and excreted by the kidneys.

metformin causes bloating and diarrhea

Prior to discharge the PN is reinforcing teaching for a client diagnosed with type 2 diabetes who has been prescribed a heart-healthy diet, metformin 1000 mg orally bid, and increased physical activity to 10,000 steps per day. Which statements by the client would alert the PN that further instruction is needed? (Select all that apply.)

A. "I will stop taking my diabetes medications if I become bloated and nauseated."
B. "I will increase my fiber and water intake."
C. "My feet are always cold, so I'll use my heating pad on the low setting."
D. "I'll continue to walk every afternoon."
E. "I'll get rid of my open-toe, open-heel shoes."

HESI Test Question Approach

Positive? YES NO

Key Words

Rephrase

Rule Out Choices

A B C D E

Other Endocrine Problems

Which client should the practical nurse collect data from first?

A. The client with hyperthyroidism who has exophthalmos
B. The client with diabetes type 1 who has an inflamed foot ulcer
C. The client with Cushing's syndrome who has moon facies
D. The client with Addison's disease who has tremors and diaphoresis

HESI Test Question Approach

Positive? YES NO

Key Words

Rephrase

Rule Out Choices

A B C D

Thyroid Gland Feedback Loop

Hypothalamus

⇩

TRH (+)

Anterior pituitary

- T_3 and T_4 (−) TSH (+)
- Thyroid gland

Hyperthyroidism   *Grave's Disease*

Nursing Assessment

- Enlarged thyroid gland
- Exophthalmos
- Weight loss
- Elevated T_3
- Elevated T_4
- Diarrhea
- Tachycardia
- Bruit over thyroid

Nursing and Collaborative Management

- Diet: high protein, high calorie, low caffeine, and low fiber
- Treatment may trigger hypothyroidism; client may need hormone replacement.
- Propylthiouracil (PTU) therapy to block the synthesis of T_3 and T_4
- Iodine (^{131}I), a radioactive therapy prescribed to destroy thyroid cells

Surgical Management

- Thyroidectomy
  - Position in high Fowler's position.
  - Check behind neck for drainage.
  - Support neck when moving client to avoid flexion of the neck.
  - Monitor for laryngeal edema (hoarseness and inability to speak).
  - Place tracheotomy set, oxygen, and suction equipment at bedside.
  - Place calcium gluconate or calcium gluceptate at bedside.

Hypothyroidism   *slow low cold and dry*

- Fatigue
- Bradycardia
- Weight gain
- Constipation
- Periorbital edema
- Cold intolerance
- Low T_3 (<70 ng/dL)
- Low T_4 (<5 ng/dL)

Nursing and Collaborative Management

- Be alert for myxedema coma, an acute exacerbation of hypothyroidism.   *cuts off airway*
- Maintain airway.

- Teach medication regimen.
- Monitor for side effects of medications.
- Monitor for signs and symptoms of constipation.

Thyroid Preparations

- Levothyroxine sodium (Eltroxin and Euthyrox)
  — Take first thing in the morning prior to food.
  — Monitor heart rate; hold for pulse >100 beats/min.
- Levothyroxine (T_4) and liothyronine (T_3; Liotrix)
  — Rapid onset

Addison's Disease   *Add a sone - need steroids*

↓Na ↑K⁺ = kidney broken

Etiology

- Sudden withdrawal from corticosteroids
- Hyposecretion of adrenal cortex hormones
- Lack of pituitary ACTH

Signs and Symptoms

- Weight loss
- Nausea and/or vomiting, anorexia
- Hypovolemia
- Hypoglycemia
- Hyponatremia
- Hyperkalemia
- Loss of body hair
- Postural hypotension
- Hyperpigmentation

Nursing and Collaborative Management

- Check vital signs frequently.
- Weigh daily.
- Monitor serum electrolytes.
- Monitor for muscle weakness.
- Monitor serum glucose.
- Diet: ↑sodium, ↓ potassium, ↑ carbohydrates
- Encourage client to drink at least 3 L of fluid per day.
- Monitor for symptoms of overdosage or underdosage of corticosteroid and mineralocorticoid therapy.
- Instruct client to carry emergency kit with 100 mg IM corticosteroid.

Cushing's Syndrome   *too much steroid = too much sugar and salt — check lungs*

watch for CBG ↑ infection

Cushing's syndrome is an excess of adrenocorticoid activity caused by adrenal, pituitary, or hypothalamus tumors. The most common cause is iatrogenic administration of exogenous corticosteroids.

Nursing Assessment

- Moon face and edema of lower extremities
- Flat affect, irritability, anxiety, depression, and psychosis
- Truncal obesity with abdominal striae
- Buffalo hump (fat deposits)
- Muscle atrophy, weakness
- Dry, pale, thin skin
- Hypertension
- Osteoporosis
- Immunosuppression
- Hirsutism
- Laboratory results

— Hyperglycemia
— Hypocalcemia
— Hypernatremia
— Hypokalemia
— Increased plasma cortisol levels

Nursing and Collaborative Management

■ Monitor for signs and symptoms of infection
— Fever
— Skin lesions
— Elevated WBCs
— Avoid extreme temperatures, infections, and emotional disturbances.
— Wear MedicAlert -or- medical bracelet.
■ Diet: ↓ sodium, ↓ carbohydrate

The PN suspects a postoperative thyroidectomy client may have had the inadvertent removal of the parathyroid gland when the client begins to experience which symptoms? (Select all that apply.) *larngeal stridor from tetany*
A. Hematoma formation
B. Harsh, vibratory sounds on inspiration and expiration
C. Tingling of lips, hands, and toes
D. Positive Chvostek's sign
E. Sensation of fullness at the incision site

HESI Test Question Approach			
Positive?		**YES**	**NO**
Key Words			
Rephrase			
Rule Out Choices			
A	B	C	D	E

The client at the assisted living facility is prescribed prednisone 10 mg orally daily. The PN reinforces teaching for the client about the medication. Which statement by the client indicates that further teaching is necessary?
A. "I can take aspirin if I need it for pain."
B. "I need to take the medication at the same time daily."
C. "I need to check for bruising on my skin."
D. "If I gain more than 5 lb a week, I will call my doctor."

HESI Test Question Approach			
Positive?		**YES**	**NO**
Key Words			
Rephrase			
Rule Out Choices			
A	B	C	D

Sexually Transmitted Infections (STIs)

■ Symptoms and treatment
— Vary by disease
■ Teach safe sex.
— Limit number of partners.
— Practice abstinence and mutual monogamy.
— Use latex condoms.
— Lifestyle risks: drugs and alcohol

- Report incidence of STIs to appropriate health agencies

Refer to the review manuals for more in-depth information about STIs:
- *Evolve Reach Comprehensive Review for the NCLEX-RN Examination* (powered by HESI)
- *Mosby's Comprehensive Review of Nursing for the NCLEX-RN Examination*
- *Saunders Comprehensive Review for the NCLEX-RN Examination*

Female Reproductive Problems

A 52-year-old client who had an abdominal hysterectomy for cervical adenocarcinoma in situ is preparing for discharge. Which recommendation should the PN offer the client about women's health and screening exams?
A. "Continue your annual Pap smear, mammogram, clinical breast exam, and monthly breast self-exam (BSE)."
B. "A Pap smear is no longer necessary, but continue your annual mammogram and clinical breast exam, plus monthly BSE."
C. "When the ovaries have been removed, only an annual mammogram and clinical breast exam are necessary."
D. "Annual mammograms are not necessary if biannual clinical breast exams and weekly BSE are done."

HESI Test Question Approach		
Positive?	YES	NO
Key Words		
Rephrase		
Rule Out Choices		
A	B	C	D

Benign Uterine Tumors
- Arise from muscle tissue of the uterus.
- Signs and symptoms
  - Menorrhagia
  - Uterine enlargement
  - Dysmenorrhea
  - Anemia secondary to menorrhagia
  - Uterine enlargement
  - Low back pain and pelvic pain
- Tend to disappear after menopause.
- Fertility issues
- Nonsurgical options
  - Magnetic resonance–guided focused ultrasound
- Surgical options
  - Myomectomy
  - Hysterectomy

A 76-year-old client reports that since she stopped hormone replacement therapy (HRT), she has had increased vaginal discomfort during intercourse. What action should the PN take?

A. Suggest that the client use a vaginal cream or lubricant.
B. Recommend that the client abstain from sexual intercourse.
C. Teach the client Kegel exercises to be performed daily.
D. Instruct the client to resume HRT.

HESI Test Question Approach			
Positive?		YES	NO
Key Words			
Rephrase			
Rule Out Choices			
A	B	C	D

Pelvic Organ Prolapse: Uterine Prolapse, Cystocele, and Rectocele

Preventive Measures

- Postpartum perineal (Kegel) exercises
- Spaced pregnancies
- Weight control
- Different signs and symptoms for each condition
- Surgical intervention
  — Hysterectomy
  — Anterior and posterior vaginal repair

Nursing and Collaborative Management

- Postoperative pain management
- Monitor postoperative urinary output.
- Observe for postoperative signs and symptoms of bleeding and infection.

A client who had a vaginal hysterectomy the previous day is saturating perineal pads with blood and requires frequent changes during the night. What priority action should the nurse take?

A. Provide iron-rich foods on each dietary tray.
B. Monitor the client's vital signs every 2 hours. *and notify MD*
C. Administer IV fluids at the prescribed rate. *can't do*
D. Encourage postoperative leg exercises.

HESI Test Question Approach			
Positive?		YES	NO
Key Words			
Rephrase			
Rule Out Choices			
A	B	C	D

Male Reproductive Problems

Etiology and Pathophysiology

Prostatitis is one of the most common male urological disorders. Common manifestations of acute bacterial prostatitis include:

- Fever and chills
- Back pain
- Perineal pain
- Dysuria
- Urinary frequency
- Urgency
- Cloudy urine

Diagnostic Studies

- Urinalysis (UA)
- Urine culture
- White blood cells (WBCs)
- Blood cultures
- PSA test (may be done to rule out prostate cancer)

Nursing and Collaborative Management

- Antibiotics
  — Sulfamethoxazole-trimethoprim suspension
  — Ciprofloxacin hydrochloride
- Antiinflammatory agents for pain control
- Encourage fluid intake

Sexual Functioning

Vasectomy is the bilateral surgical ligation of the vas deferens performed for the purpose of sterilization.

Erectile dysfunction (ED) is the inability to attain or maintain an erect penis to allow satisfactory sexual performance. ED is increasing in all segments of the sexually active male population. ED can result from a number of factors, including:

- Diabetes
- Vascular disease (most common cause)
- Side effects of medications
- Result of surgery (prostatectomy)
- Trauma
- Chronic illness
- Decreased gonadal hormone secretion
- Stress
- Depression

The treatment for ED is based on the underlying cause.

Oral Drug Therapy Example

- Sildenafil citrate
- Dosage: PO 25 to 100 mg, 1 dose per day, 1 hour before sexual activity
- These drugs may potentiate the hypotensive effect of nitrates; they are contraindicated for individuals taking nitrates (e.g., nitroglycerin).
- Teach clients to seek medical attention for an erection lasting longer than 4 hours (priapism).
- Use with caution in the elderly as drugs are slow to metabolize and to be excreted.

8

Movement, Coordination, and Sensory Input *Musculo skeletal etc*

The PN initiates neuro checks for a client at risk for neurological compromise. Which manifestation typically provides the first indication of altered neurological function?
A. Change in level of consciousness
B. Increasing muscular weakness
C. Changes in pupil size bilaterally
D. Progressive nuchal rigidity

HESI Test Question Approach			
Positive?		YES	NO
Key Words			
Rephrase			
Rule Out Choices			
A	**B**	**C**	**D**

Altered State of Consciousness

Glasgow Coma Scale

- Used to assess level of consciousness (LOC)
- Score: maximum, 15; minimum, 3
  - ≤ 7 = Coma
  - 3 to 4 = High mortality rate
  - > 8 = Good prognosis
- A decrease in LOC may be the earliest sign of increasing intracranial pressure (ICP).
- Neurological vital signs
  - Pupil size (with sizing scale)
  - Limb movement (with scale)
  - Vital signs (blood pressure, temperature, pulse, and respirations)

Nursing Assessment

- Assess for early signs and symptoms of changes in LOC
  - Decreasing LOC (most sensitive indicator)
  - Change in orientation
- Late signs
  - Cushing's triad (emergency)
    - Widening pulse pressure
    - Slowing heart rate; full bounding pulse
    - Slowing and irregular respirations
  - Change in size, response of pupils; dilated on side of injury initially
  - Elevated temperature
  - Posturing
- Assess for change in respiratory status
  - Cheyne-Stokes respiration

Nursing and Collaborative Management

- Maintain airway and provide adequate oxygenation.
  - Mechanical ventilation is possible with ↓ LOC.

GLASGOW COMA SCALE*	
Eye Opening	
Spontaneous	4
To sound	3
To pain	2
Never	1
Motor Response	
Obeys commands	6
Localizes pain	5
Normal flexion (withdrawal)	4
Abnormal flexion	3
Extension	2
None	1
Verbal Response	
Oriented	5
Confused conversation	4
Inappropriate words	3
Incomprehensible sounds	2
None	1

* The highest possible score is 15

— Hyperventilate before suctioning.
— Limit suctioning to 15 seconds.
— Keep airway free of secretions.
— Prevent aspiration: Turn head to side.
- Prevent complications related to sustained ↑ ICP.
   — ICP monitoring target: 5 to 15 mm Hg
   — Elevate head of bed to 30 to 45 degrees to promote venous return.
   — Place the neck in a neutral position (not flexed or extended) to promote venous drainage.
   — Position client to avoid flexion of the hips, waist, and neck and rotation of the head, especially to the right.
   — Implement measures to help client avoid Valsalva maneuver.

Medications
- Hyperosmotic agents
   — 20% mannitol via a filtered tubing
   — Steroids increase the risk for infections.
     • Decadron
     • Solu-Medrol
- Prophylactic phenytoin (Dilantin)
- Barbiturates used to induce coma when ICP can't otherwise be controlled.
   — Prophylactic levetiracetam (Keppra)
   — Nembutal (Novopentobarb [Canada])
- Diuretics
   — Alternate with mannitol
- Avoid narcotics.

Which change in the status of a client being treated for increased ICP warrants immediate action by the PN?
A. Urinary output increases from 20 to 50 mL/hr.
B. Arterial Po₂ increases from 80 to 90 mm Hg.
C. Glasgow Coma Scale score changes from 5 to 7.
D. Pulse drops from 88 to 68 beats/min.

HESI Test Question Approach			
Positive?		YES	NO
Key Words			
Rephrase			
Rule Out Choices			
A	B	C	D

Head Injury
Nursing Assessment

- Changes in LOC
- Signs of increased ICP
  - Changes in VS
  - Headache, amnesia, and personality changes
  - Vomiting
  - Pupillary changes: unequal, dilated
  - Seizure
  - Ataxia
  - Abnormal posturing (decerebrate or decorticate)
  - Extremity motor strength and use
  - Check for lacerations, bruises, skull depression, confusion, combativeness

CSF Leakage

- Risk of meningitis with leakage
- Usual signs of increased ICP may not be seen with CSF leakage as the pressure can be relieved by the leak.
- Drainage may come from nose (rhinorrhea) or ears (otorrhea).

Nursing and Collaborative Management

- Neurological assessment every 15 min
- Notify healthcare provider at **first** sign of deterioration.
- Limit visitors.
- Keep room quiet.
- Prevent straining.
- Keep HOB at 30 to 45 degrees unless BP significantly lowered.
- Avoid neck flexion/straining.
- Monitor I & O.

The PN is assisting with a class on stroke prevention for clients with hypertension. What information is most important to provide the clients in the class?
A. Salt restriction diet
B. Weight reduction
C. Medication compliance
D. Risk for stroke

HESI Test Question Approach			
Positive?		YES	NO
Key Words			
Rephrase			
Rule Out Choices			
A	B	C	D

During the evaluation, which assessments indicate a late sign of increased ICP for a client newly diagnosed with a head injury? (Select all that apply.)
A. Alteration in the ability to respond to questions
B. Alteration in the ability to swallow liquids
C. Consensual response of pupils
D. Heart rate, 50; BP, 192/60
E. Drooping of the mouth on one side

HESI Test Question Approach				
Positive?			YES	NO
Key Words				
Rephrase				
Rule Out Choices				
A	B	C	D	E

Stroke (Brain Attack) or Cerebrovascular Accident

- Hemorrhage into brain tissue (medical emergency)
- Ischemic clot
  - Thrombotic
  - Embolic
- Transient ischemic attack (TIA)
  - Temporary episode of neurological dysfunction lasting less than 24 hours and often less than 15 minutes (Most fully resolve.)

Nursing and Collaborative Management

- Time lost is brain lost FAST.
- Hemorrhagic or ischemic
- CT scan or MRI
- Prepare for thrombolytic (limited therapeutic window).
- Assess for signs and symptoms of increased ICP.
- Assess verbal ability and plan care appropriate to client's ability to communicate.
- Assess swallowing to prevent aspiration.
- Assess for bowel and bladder control.
- Assess functional abilities.
  - Mobility
  - Activities of daily living (ADLs)
  - Elimination: Prevent distention to avoid impairing respirations.

A client with Parkinson's disease is prescribed carbidopa-levodopa. Which observation by the PN indicates that the desired effect of the medication is being achieved?

A. Decreased blood pressure
B. Steady gait
C. Increased salivation
D. Increased attention span

Parkinson's Disease

- Symptoms
  - Rigidity
  - Mask-like face
  - Akinesia
    - Difficulty initiating and continuing movement
  - Tremors
    - Resting tremors
    - Pill rolling
  - Postural instability

Nursing Plans and Interventions

- SAFETY is always a priority!
- Take medications with meals; administer promptly.
- Change positions slowly to reduce postural hypotension.
- Thicken liquids.
- Soft, ground foods
- Encourage activity and exercise.

Medications

- Dopaminergics
  - Levodopa (L-dopa and dopamine)
    - Blocks breakdown of levodopa to allow more levodopa to cross the blood-brain barrier
    - Avoid foods high in vitamin B_6 and protein.
  - Carbidopa-levodopa (Sinemet; Parcopa [orally dissolving tablet])
  - Allows for less use of levodopa and helps ↓ side effects.
- Dopaminergic agonists
  - Rotigotine (Neupro) Pramipexole (Mirapex)
  - Ropinirole hydrochloride (Requip)
  - Amantadine (Symmetrel)
  - Apomorphine (Apokyn)
- Anticholinergics treat tremors; use with caution in older adults due to side effects.
  - Trihexyphenidyl (Trihexyphen [Canada]; Artane)
  - Benztropine mesylate (Cogentin)
  - Procyclidine hydrochloride (Akineton; Kemadrin)

- Antihistamine - Diphenhydramine (Benadryl)
- Monoamine oxidase inhibitors: Selegiline hydrochloride (Anipryl [Canada], Eldepryl)
- Catechol-O-methyl transferase (COMT) inhibitors Entacapone (Comtan)

Guillain-Barré Syndrome

- Usually occurs after upper respiratory or gastrointestinal infection.
- Ascending paralysis
- Rapid demyelination of nerves
- Paralysis of respiratory system may occur quickly.
- Prepare to intubate.
- Some patients experience a prolonged recovery time.

Treatment

- Plasmapheresis over 10 to 15 days
- IV high-dose immunoglobulin (Sandoglobulin) is as effective as plasma exchange and has the advantage of immediate availability and greater safety. Clients receiving high-dose immunoglobulin must be well hydrated and have adequate renal function.
- Maintain patent airway.
- Reposition frequently; assess range of motion until patient regains use of extremities.
- Impaired swallowing may require TPN; NPO if gag reflex is absent.
- Supervise small, frequent feedings; thicken liquids.

Multiple Sclerosis (MS)

- Demyelination of the central nervous system (CNS) myelin
- Messages are garbled and short-circuited from brain to CNS.
- Disease is characterized by periods of remission and exacerbation.
- Assessment findings
  — Changes in visual field: diplopia and scotomas
  — Weaknesses are in extremities.
  — Numbness
  — Visual or swallowing difficulties
  — Severe fatigue and emotional problems
  — Gait disturbances

Nursing and Collaborative Management

- Avoid abrupt changes in room lighting.
- Provide assistive devices to meet the patient's specific deficits.
- Thicken liquids.

Medication Management

Focuses on controlling symptoms
- Corticosteroids to treat acute exacerbations by reducing edema and inflammation
  — ACTH, prednisone, and methylprednisolone
- Immunomodulators to prevent relapses
  — Interferon beta (Betaseron, Avonex, Rebif)
  — Glatiramer acetate (Copaxone) ↑ risk for allergic and/or anaphylactic reaction.

- Immunosuppressants
  — Mitoxantrone (Novantrone)
- Cholinergics
  — Bethanechol (Urecholine)
  — Neostigmine (Prostigmin)
- Anticholinergics to treat bladder spasms
  — Propantheline (Pro-Banthine)
  — Oxybutynin (Ditropan)
- Muscle relaxants to treat spasticity
  — Diazepam (Valium)
  — Baclofen (Lioresal)
  — Dantrolene (Dantrium)
  — Tizanidine (Zanaflex)
- CNS stimulants to treat fatigue
  — Pemoline (Cylert)
  — Methylphenidate (Ritalin)
  — Modafinil (Provigil)
- Antiviral/antiparkinsonian drugs to treat fatigue
  — Amantadine (Symmetrel)

Myasthenia Gravis
- Chronic neuromuscular autoimmune disease
- Causes fluctuating weakness and abnormal fatigue of voluntary muscles, which increase throughout the day.

Nursing Assessment
- Ocular muscle weakness; difficulty keeping eyes opened or closed
- Bulbar muscle weakness; difficulty speaking, swallowing, or chewing
- Skeletal muscle weakness, primarily central muscles, fatigue, and loss of bowel and bladder control

Diagnosis
- Based on clinical presentation and history
  — Muscle weakness
- Confirmed by improved response to anticholinesterase drugs, edrophonium (Enlon, Tensilon) test; is given in small doses over 15-45 seconds.

Medications
- Anticholinesterase agents
  — To achieve maximum strength and endurance
  — Block action of cholinesterase
  — Increase levels of ACh at junctions
  — Common medications: mestinon, prostigmin
    - Start with minimal doses.
    - Onset: 30 min
    - Duration: 3 to 4 hours
    - Must take on time!
- Corticosteroids
  — Prednisone
- Immunosuppressants
  — Azathioprine (Imuran)
  — Cyclophosphamide (Cytoxan)

Types of Crisis
- Myasthenic
  — Medical emergency

— Neostigmine (Prostigmin) may be administered.
— Caused by under medicating or infection
— Positive Tensilon test
— Changes in VS, cyanosis, loss of cough and gag reflex, and incontinence
— May require intubation.
■ Cholinergic
— Atropine may be administered.
— Results from overmedication and toxic levels of anticholinesterase medications.
— Negative Tensilon test
— Symptoms: abdominal cramps, diarrhea, and excessive pulmonary secretions

Nursing Interventions
■ Coughing and deep-breathing exercises
■ Suction equipment at bedside
■ Sit upright when eating and for 1 hour afterward.
■ Keep chin downward when swallowing.
■ Plan activities and rest carefully; weakness is greater at the end of the day.

Spinal Cord Injury
■ Injuries classified by
— Extent of injury: complete vs. incomplete
— Level of injury: skeletal and neurologic
— Mechanism of injury; example is flexion.
■ Injuries classified as complete or incomplete
— Transection/partial transection
■ Rule of thumb
— Injury above C8 = quadriplegic/tetraplegia
— Injury below C8 = paraplegic

Nursing Assessment
■ Start with ABCs; priority nursing assessment.
■ Determine quality of respiratory status.
■ Check neurological status.
■ Assess vital signs.
■ Hypotension and bradycardia can occur with injuries above T6.

Nursing Plans and Interventions
■ Immobilize and stabilize!
■ Keep neck and body in anatomical alignment.
■ Maintain patent airway.
■ Clients with cervical injuries are placed in skeletal traction.
■ High-dose corticosteroids are used to control edema during first 24 hours.
■ Spinal shock: temporary loss of sensation and reflexes, usually within first 48 hours
■ Flaccid paralysis: neurogenic shock
— Complete loss of reflexes
— Hypotension
— Bradycardia; treat with atropine sulfate.
— Bowel and bladder distention, paralytic ileus with 72 hours of trauma
— Reverse as quickly as possible.

- Autonomic dysreflexia
  — Medical emergency that occurs in clients with injuries at or above T6
  — Exaggerated autonomic reflex response
  — Usually triggered by bowel or bladder distention
  — Signs and symptoms: severe headache, ↑ BP, bradycardia, and profuse sweating
  — Elevate head of bed (while maintaining correct alignment); relieve bowel or bladder distention.
  — Notify HCP immediately.

Rehabilitation

- Assess for paralytic ileus.
  — Assess bowel sounds.
- Kinetic bed to promote blood flow, ROM exercises
- Antiembolic stockings, sequential compression devices
- Protect from skin breakdown.
- Psychosocial assessments
- Bowel and bladder training
  — Keep bladder empty and urine dilute and acidic to help prevent urinary tract infection, a common cause of death after spinal cord injury.

The PN is caring for a client hospitalized with Guillain-Barré syndrome. Which information would be most important for the PN to report to the RN?
A. Ascending numbness from feet to knees
B. Decrease in cognitive status
C. Blurred vision and sensation changes
D. Persistent unilateral headache

HESI Test Question Approach			
Positive?		YES	NO
Key Words			
Rephrase			
Rule Out Choices			
A	B	C	D

Which action by the unlicensed assistive personnel (UAP) requires immediate follow-up by the nurse?
A. Positions a client who is 12 hours post above-the-knee amputation (AKA) with the residual limb elevated on a pillow.
B. Assists a client with ambulation while the client uses a cane on the unaffected side.
C. Accompanies a client who has lupus erythematosus to sit outside in the sun during a break.
D. Helps a client with rheumatoid arthritis to the bathroom after the client takes Celebrex.

HESI Test Question Approach			
Positive?		YES	NO
Key Words			
Rephrase			
Rule Out Choices			
A	B	C	D

Fractures

Signs and Symptoms
- Pain, swelling, and deformity of the extremity
- Discoloration, loss of functional ability
- Fracture generally evident on x-ray study.

Nursing and Collaborative Management
- Instruct client on proper use of assistive devices.
- Assess for 5 Ps of neurovascular functioning.
  - Pain
  - Paresthesia
  - Pulse
  - Pallor
  - Paralysis
- Assess neurovascular area distal to injury.
  - Skin color, temperature, sensation, capillary refill, mobility, pain, pulses, and acute compartment syndrome

Treatment
- Closed reduction without incision
- Open reduction with incision
- Postreduction
  - Cast, special handling while still wet
  - Traction, continuous or intermittent
  - External fixation
  - Splints
  - Orthoses (braces)

An adult client with a fracture of the femur is being discharged from the fast-track clinic after application of a plaster cast. The PN should reinforce with the client the need to use which method to dry the cast over the next 24 hours?
A. Place plastic wrap on the bottom of the cast to prevent sticking.
B. Support the cast on a firm surface during the night.
C. Keep the cast's surfaces exposed to circulating air.
D. Use a blow dryer set at low for 10 minutes every hour for four hours.

HESI Test Question Approach		
Positive?	YES	NO
Key Words		
Rephrase		
Rule Out Choices		
A	B	C	D

Joint Replacement
- After surgery
  - Check circulation, sensation, and movement of extremity distal to replacement area.
  - Maintain body in proper alignment.
  - Encourage fluid intake.
  - Have client use bedpan or commode chair.
  - Coordinate rehabilitation process.
- Discharge home
  - Safety
  - Accessibility

- Drugs
  — Anticoagulants
  — Analgesics
  — Parenteral antibiotics

Amputation
- Postoperative care
  — Monitor surgical dressing for drainage.
  — Ensure proper body alignment.
  — Elevate residual limb (stump) for first 24 hours.
  — Do NOT elevate after 48 hours.
  — Provide passive range of motion (ROM) and encourage prone position periodically to reduce risk of contracture.
  — Perform proper stump bandaging to prepare for prosthesis.
  — Coordinate care with OT and PT and SW.

Remember: Phantom limb pain is real and requires pharmacological interventions.
Assess and address grieving.

A postmenopausal woman with a BMI of 19 has come to the clinic for her annual well-woman examination. Which teaching plan topic is most important for the nurse to prepare for this high-risk client?
A. Osteoporosis
B. Obesity
C. Anorexia
D. Breast cancer

HESI Test Question Approach		
Positive?	**YES**	**NO**
Key Words		
Rephrase		
Rule Out Choices		
A	B	C	D

Osteoporosis
Risk Factors
- Small-boned, postmenopausal females, Caucasian, Asian, pregnancy, breastfeeding, plus family history
- Diet low in calcium
- Excessive use of alcohol, tobacco, and caffeine
- Inactive or sedentary lifestyle
- Men: low testosterone level

Nursing Assessment
- Dowager hump
- Kyphosis of the dorsal spine
- Loss of height
- Pathological fractures
- Compression fracture of spine can occur.

Nursing and Collaborative Management
- Keep bed in low position.
- Provide adequate lighting.
- Avoid using throw rugs.

- Provide assistance with ambulation.
- Follow regular exercise program.
- Diet high in vitamin D, protein, and calcium
- 20 minutes of UV exposure per day
- Routine DEXA screening begins at 60.

Osteoporosis Drug Therapy
- Bisphosphonates
  - Alendronate (Fosamax)
  - Ibandronate (Boniva)
  - Pamidronate (Aredia)
  - Risedronate (Actonel)
- Selective estrogen receptor modulators
  - Raloxifene (Evista)
  - Teriparatide (Forteo)

Rheumatoid Arthritis
- Chronic, systemic, progressive deterioration of connective tissue
- Etiology is unknown but believed to be autoimmune.

Nursing Assessment
- Affects young to middle age.
- Affects females > males.
- Systemic, with exacerbations and remissions
- Affects small joints first and then spreads.
- Stiffness (May decrease with use.)
- Decreased range of motion
- Joint pain
- Elevated erythrocyte sedimentation rate (ESR)
- Positive rheumatoid factor (RF) in 80% of clients
- Narrowed joint space

Nursing and Collaborative Management
- Drug therapy:
  - High-dose ASA or NSAIDs
  - Systemic corticosteroids
  - Disease-modifying antirheumatic drugs
    - Methotrexate (Rheumatrex)
    - Sulfasalazine (Azulfidine)
    - Hydroxychloroquine (Plaquenil)
    - Leflunomide (Arava)
- Heat and cold applications
- Weight management if indicated
- Rest and joint protection to maintain function
- Assistive devices
  - Shower chair
  - Canes, walkers
  - Straight-backed chairs with arms and elevated seats

Lupus Erythematosus
- Discoid lupus erythematosus (DLE) affects skin only.
- Systemic lupus erythematosus (SLE) is more prevalent than DLE.
- Major trigger factors
  - Sunlight
  - Infectious agents
  - Stress
  - Drugs
  - Pregnancy

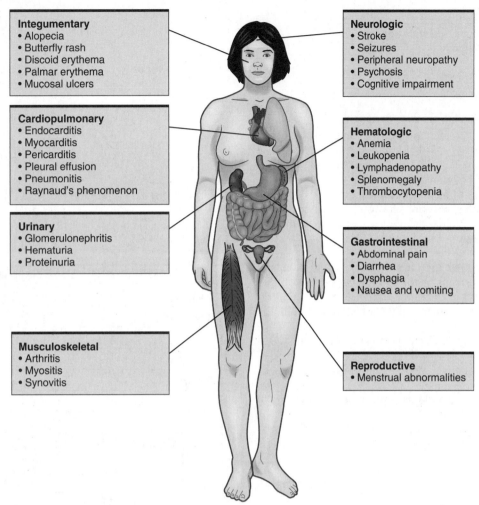

Integumentary
- Alopecia
- Butterfly rash
- Discoid erythema
- Palmar erythema
- Mucosal ulcers

Neurologic
- Stroke
- Seizures
- Peripheral neuropathy
- Psychosis
- Cognitive impairment

Cardiopulmonary
- Endocarditis
- Myocarditis
- Pericarditis
- Pleural effusion
- Pneumonitis
- Raynaud's phenomenon

Hematologic
- Anemia
- Leukopenia
- Lymphadenopathy
- Splenomegaly
- Thrombocytopenia

Urinary
- Glomerulonephritis
- Hematuria
- Proteinuria

Gastrointestinal
- Abdominal pain
- Diarrhea
- Dysphagia
- Nausea and vomiting

Musculoskeletal
- Arthritis
- Myositis
- Synovitis

Reproductive
- Menstrual abnormalities

Fig. 8-1 Multisystem involvement in systemic lupus erythematosus. (Lewis, S., Dirksen, S., Heitkemper, M., Bucher, L. (2014). *Medical-surgical nursing: Assessment and management of clinical problems* (9th ed.). St. Louis: Mosby. Fig. 65-9, p. 1583.)

Nursing Assessment
- DLE: scaly rash and/or butterfly rash over bridge of nose
- SLE: joint pain, fever, nephritis, and pericarditis (See Fig. 8-1.)
- Photosensitivity

Nursing and Collaborative Management
- Teaching
  — Drugs
  — Pain management
  — Disease process
  — Conservation of energy
  — Avoid exposure to ultraviolet rays.
  — Avoid and/or reduce stress.
  — Use mild soaps and creams for skin care.
  — Use steroids for joint inflammation.
- Therapeutic exercise and heat therapy
- Pregnancy counseling

Degenerative Joint Disease (Osteoarthritis)

- Joint pain increases with activity
- Morning stiffness
- Crepitus
- Limited movement
- Joint enlargement

Nursing and Collaborative Management

- Follow weight-reduction diet if indicated.
- Excessive use of involved joint may accelerate degeneration.
- Use proper body mechanics.
- Keep joints in functional position.
- Hot and cold applications for pain and stiffness
- NSAIDs, opioid analgesics, and intraarticular corticosteroids

The PN observes an elderly client with glaucoma administer eye drops by tilting his head back, instilling each drop close to the inner canthus, and keeping his eye closed for 15 seconds. What action should the PN take first?

A. Ask the client whether another family member is available to administer the drops.

B. Review the correct steps of the procedure with the client.

C. Administer the eye drops correctly in the other eye to demonstrate the technique.

D. Discuss the importance of correct eye drop administration for individuals with glaucoma.

HESI Test Question Approach		
Positive?	**YES**	**NO**
Key Words		
Rephrase		
Rule Out Choices		
A	**B**	**C**	**D**

Glaucoma

- Primary open-angle glaucoma more common
  - Drainage channels become clogged.
  - Aqueous humor flow is reduced in trabecular meshwork.
- Primary closed-angle glaucoma painful if acute
  - Bulging lens from age-related processes disrupts flow.
- Silent thief of vision
- Normally painless until later stages
- Loss of peripheral vision
- May see halos around lights.
- Diagnosed with eye examination
  - Tonometer used to measure intraocular pressure.

Nursing Plans and Interventions

- Keys to treatment
  - ↓ Intraocular pressure; normal is 10 to 21 mm Hg.
  - ↓ Aqueous humor production
  - ↑ Drainage of aqueous humor
  - Teach client and family proper eye-drop instillation.
  - Teach client how to avoid activities that can increase intraocular pressure.

Nursing Management and Collaborative Therapy

- Ambulatory/home care for open-angle glaucoma
  — Drug therapy
    - β-Adrenergic blockers
    - α-Adrenergic agonists
    - Cholinergic agents decrease visual acuity in low-light environments.
    - Carbonic anhydrase inhibitors
  — Surgical options
    - Argon laser trabeculoplasty
    - Trabeculectomy with or without filtering implant
- Acute care for closed-angle glaucoma
  — Topical cholinergic agent
  — Hyperosmotic agent
  — Laser peripheral iridotomy
  — Surgical iridectomy

Glaucoma Drug Therapy

- β-Adrenergic blockers
  — Betaxolol (Betoptic)
  — Metipranolol (OptiPranolol)
  — Timolol maleate (Timoptic, Istalol)
- α-Adrenergic agonists
  — Dipivefrin (Propine)
  — Epinephrine (Epifrin, Eppy, Gaucon, Epinal, Eppy/N)
  — Brimonidine (Alphagan)
  — Latanoprost (Xalatan)
- Cholinergic agents (miotics)
  — Carbachol (Isopto Carbachol)
  — Pilocarpine (Akarpine; Isopto-Carpine, Pilocar, Pilopine, Piloptic, and Pilostat)
- Carbonic anhydrase inhibitors
  — Systemic
    - Acetazolamide (Diamox)
    - Dichlorphenamide (Daranide)
  — Topical
    - Brinzolamide (Azopt)
    - Dorzolamide (Trusopt)
- Combination therapy
  — Timolol maleate and dorzolamide (Cosopt)
- Hyperosmolar agents
  — Glycerin liquid (Ophthalgan and Osmoglyn Oral)
  — Isosorbide solution (Ismotic)
  — Mannitol solution (Osmitrol)

Cataracts

- Clouding or opacity of the lens d/t trauma, aging or congenital defect
- Early signs
  — Blurred vision
  — Decreased color perception
- Late signs
  — Double vision
  — Clouded pupil

Nursing and Collaborative Management

- Preoperative
  - Assess current medications being taken.
  - Stop anticoagulants before surgery.
  - Teach client how to instill eye drops.
- Postoperative
  - Wear eye shield while sleeping.
  - Avoid lifting >10 lb.
  - Avoid lying on operative side and Valsalva maneuver.
  - Report signs of increased intraocular pressure.
    - Acute pain is an abnormal finding. Pain generally is treated with acetaminophen.
    - Loss of peripheral vision
    - Visual field defects

Eye Trauma/Injury

- Trauma
  - Determine type of injury.
  - Early notification of HCP to preserve vision
  - Position client in sitting position to reduce intraocular pressure.
  - Never attempt to remove embedded object.
  - Irrigate eye if a chemical injury has occurred.
- Detached retina
  - Described as a curtain falling over the visual field
  - Sudden loss of vision
  - Painless
  - Client may see black spots or floaters (indicates bleeding has occurred with detachment).
  - Retina is repaired surgically.
  - Keep eye patch over affected area.

Hearing Loss

- Conductive hearing loss
  - Sounds do not travel to the inner ear.
  - Client may benefit from hearing aid.
- Sensorineural hearing loss
  - Sound distorted by defect in inner ear
- Common causes
  - Infection
  - Ototoxic drugs
    - Gentamicin
    - Vancomycin
    - Furosemide
  - Trauma
  - Aging
- Assessment
  - Inability to hear whisper from 1 to 2 feet
  - Shouting in conversations
  - Turning head to favor one ear
  - Loud volume on TV

9 Pediatric Nursing

The PN directs the unlicensed assistive personnel (UAP) to play with a 4-year-old child on bed rest. Which activity or activities should the PN recommend? (Select all that apply.)
A. Monopoly board game
B. Checkers
C. 50-piece puzzle
D. Hand puppets
E. Coloring book

<table>
<tr><td colspan="3">HESI Test Question Approach</td></tr>
<tr><td>Positive?</td><td>YES</td><td>NO</td></tr>
<tr><td colspan="3">Key Words</td></tr>
<tr><td colspan="3"></td></tr>
<tr><td colspan="3"></td></tr>
<tr><td colspan="3">Rephrase</td></tr>
<tr><td colspan="3"></td></tr>
<tr><td colspan="3"></td></tr>
<tr><td colspan="3">Rule Out Choices</td></tr>
<tr><td>A</td><td>B</td><td>C</td><td>D</td><td>E</td></tr>
</table>

Growth and Development

Know the norms for growth and development!

- Infant
  - Doubles birth weight by 6 months and triples by 12 months
  - Sits upright without support by 8 months.
  - Stranger anxiety begins at 6 to 8 months.
  - Develops fine pincer grasp by 10 to 12 months.
  - Walks with support 11 months to 1 year.
  - Few words plus *mama* and *dada* at 12 months
- Toddler (1 to 3 years)
  - Produces two- to three-word sentences at 2 years
  - Begins toilet training around 2 years.
  - Ritualistic
  - No concept of time
  - Frequent tantrums
- Preschool-age child (3 to 5 years)
  - Favorite word is *Why?*
  - Can construct sentences of five to eight words.
- School-age child (6 to 12 years)
  - Each year the child gains 4 to 6 lb, grows 2 inches.
  - Learns to tell time.
  - Socialization with peers is important.
- Adolescent (12 to 19 years)
  - Rapid growth, second only to first year of life
  - Develops secondary sex characteristics.

While receiving IV antibiotics for sepsis, a 2-month-old infant is crying inconsolably, despite the mother's presence. The PN recognizes that the infant is exhibiting symptoms related to which likely condition?

A. Allergic reaction to antibiotics
B. Pain related to IV infiltration
C. Separation anxiety from mother ✗
D. Hunger and thirst ✗

HESI Test Question Approach			
Positive?		**YES**	**NO**
Key Words			
Rephrase			
Rule Out Choices			
A	**B**	**C**	**D**

Pain Assessment and Management

- Assessment based on verbal and nonverbal cues from child and includes parents' information
- Use appropriate pain scales.
- Safety is a major priority for administering medication.
- Make sure dose is safe for child's age and weight.

Immunization Teaching

- The presence of a minor illness such as the common cold does not contraindicate immunization. In general, a severe febrile illness is a contraindication.
- A fever <38.9°C (<102°F) and redness and soreness at the injection site are normal for 2 to 3 days after vaccination.
- Call physician if high-pitched crying, seizures, or high fever occur.
- *Consult immunization chart regarding immunizations (https://www.cdc.gov/vaccines/schedules/index.html)*

NOTE: Withhold MMR vaccine if client has a history of anaphylactic reaction to neomycin or eggs.

Example: Which vaccines would the nurse expect to be prescribed for a 2-month-old brought into the pediatrician's office for a well-baby checkup?

Answer: DTaP, HepB, HIB, IPV, and PCV

Communicable Diseases

The incidence of common childhood communicable diseases has declined greatly since the advent of immunizations, but they do occur, and nurses should be able to identify such infections, including:

- Measles
- Rubeola
- Rubella
- Roseola
- Mumps
- Pertussis
- Diphtheria
- Varicella

- Erythema infectiosum (fifth disease)
  — Treat fever caused by infection with acetaminophen, not ASA (acetylsalicylic acid or aspirin).
  — Isolation is required during infectious phase.
  — Teaching is the primary intervention for preventing the spread of disease; stress good handwashing.
  — Provide supportive measures until the disease runs its course.

Poisonings

- Frequent cause of childhood injury; teach poison-proofing methods for the home!
- Occurs most frequently in children less than age 6; usual peak occurs at age 2
- GI disturbance is common symptom.
- Caustic poisonings cause burns of the mouth and pharynx.
- Identify poisonous agent quickly!
- Assess ABCs
- Teach parents NOT to make the child vomit, which may cause more damage.
- Call the Poison Control Center or 911, depending on how the child is acting.

The PN is caring for a 2-year-old child suspected of having croup. What early signs of respiratory distress require immediate reporting?
A. Cyanosis
B. Restlessness
C. Crying
D. Barking cough

HESI Test Question Approach			
Positive?		YES	NO
Key Words			
Rephrase			
Rule Out Choices			
A	B	C	D

Respiratory Disorders

A 4-year-old is brought to the clinic with a fever of 103°F, a sore throat, and moderate respiratory distress caused by a suspected bacterial infection. Which medical diagnosis is contraindicated to obtaining a throat culture in the child?
A. Tonsillitis
B. Streptococcal infection
C. Bronchiolitis
D. Epiglottitis

HESI Test Question Approach			
Positive?		YES	NO
Key Words			
Rephrase			
Rule Out Choices			
A	B	C	D

A PN is caring for a child who had a tonsillectomy 2 hours ago. Which should alert the nurse that the child is bleeding?

A. Decrease in pulse
B. Increase in blood pressure
C. Frequent swallowing
D. Nasal congestion

HESI Test Question Approach			
Positive?		**YES**	**NO**
Key Words			
Rephrase			
Rule Out Choices			
A	**B**	**C**	**D**

Common Respiratory Disorders

- Be familiar with normal values for respiratory and pulse rates for children.
- Know cardinal and other signs of respiratory distress.
- Respiratory failure usually occurs before cardiac failure.

Pulmonary Infections

- Nasopharyngitis
- Tonsillitis
  - May be viral or bacterial.
  - Check prothrombin time (PT) and partial thromboplastin time (PTT) before surgery.
  - Monitor for bleeding.
  - Highest risk for bleeding is during first 24 hours and 5 to 10 days postoperative.
- Otitis media
  - Signs and symptoms: fever and pulling at ear
  - Discharge from ear
  - Administer antibiotics if prescribed.
  - Position on affected side.
  - Reduce temperature to prevent seizures.
- Bronchitis: inflammation of trachea and bronchi, rhinitis and cough, crackles and rhonchi on auscultation and symptomatic treatment
- Respiratory syncytial virus (RSV) bronchiolitis
  - Isolate the child (contact isolation).
  - Monitor respiratory status; maintain patent airway.
  - Administer antiviral agent (ribavirin aerosols, prophylactic palivizumab for high-risk children age <2 years)
- Epiglottitis
  - Signs and symptoms: high fever, sore throat, muffled voice, tripod position, and drooling
  - IV antibiotics
  - Do not examine throat; may cause complete airway obstruction.
  - Be prepared for tracheostomy.

Asthma

- Leading cause of chronic illness in children
- Allergies influence persistence and severity.

Nursing and Collaborative Management

- Signs and symptoms: tight cough, expiratory wheezing, and decreased peak flow levels
- Monitor for respiratory distress and the need for O_2 nebulizer therapy.
- Reinforce education on use of peak flow meter, nebulization treatments, and multidose inhalers.
- Rescue versus maintenance medications
- Refer to section on drug therapy for asthma and COPD in Chapter 5.

The PN is reinforcing teaching for a school-age child and the child's parent regarding the administration of inhaled betamethasone dipropionate and albuterol for the treatment of asthma. Which statement by the parent indicates that teaching has been effective?
A. "I'll keep the inhalers in the refrigerator."
B. "We only need to use the inhalers when the peak flow numbers are in the red."
C. "We will take the bronchodilator first and then the corticosteroid."
D. "I will take the corticosteroid first, wait a few minutes, and then take the bronchodilator."

HESI Test Question Approach			
Positive?		**YES**	**NO**
Key Words			
Rephrase			
Rule Out Choices			
A	**B**	**C**	**D**

The PN is reinforcing discharge teaching for parents of a 4-year-old with cystic fibrosis. Which statement by the parents demonstrates understanding of the teaching presented?
A. "We will discourage the child from playing outdoors."
B. "We will use pancreatic enzymes only if needed."
C. "We will thoroughly wash his hands when toileting."
D. "We will schedule a physical therapist evaluation."

HESI Test Question Approach			
Positive?		**YES**	**NO**
Key Words			
Rephrase			
Rule Out Choices			
A	**B**	**C**	**D**

Cystic Fibrosis (CF)

- Most common inherited disease of Caucasian children
- Diagnosis may be based on a number of criteria:
  - Chronic multisystem disorder
  - Abnormally thick mucus; primarily lungs and pancreatic involvement
  - Absence of pancreatic enzymes
  - Steatorrhea
  - Positive newborn screening test
  - First sign may be meconium ileus at birth.
  - High sweat chloride concentration (pilocarpine test or sweat test)
  - Delayed growth; poor weight gain

Nursing and Collaborative Management
- Pancreatic enzymes with each meal and snacks; fat-soluble vitamins
- Teach family percussion and postural drainage techniques.

Cardiovascular Disorders

Congenital Heart Disorders
- For description and illustrations of congenital heart disorders, see a pediatric textbook or an NCLEX review book.

Congestive Heart Failure
- Common complication of congenital heart disorders
- Early signs and symptoms: longer period for feeding, may fail to gain weight, and may be irritable and fatigued
- Later signs and symptoms: pedal edema, neck vein distention, cyanosis, tachycardia, tachypnea, coughing, retractions, wheezing, and grunting

Nursing and Collaborative Management
- Monitor vital signs, elevate head of bed, and administer O_2.
- Weigh daily on same scale.
- Digoxin, diuretics, and ACE inhibitors

Digoxin Precautions
- Count apical rate when child is at rest; withhold medication if pulse is
  - <90 to 110 beats/min as a general rule. Drug not given if pulse is below 90 to 110 beats/min in infants and young children or below 70 beats/min in older children (The cutoff point for adults is 60 beats/min.). Because pulse rate varies in children in different age groups, the written drug order should specify at what heart rate the drug is withheld.
  - Notify healthcare provider if pulse is below these rates.
- Do not skip or try to make up doses.
- Give 1 to 2 hours before meals.
- Watch for signs and symptoms of toxicity and teach them to parents:
  - Vomiting, anorexia, diarrhea, muscle weakness, and drowsiness
- Provide adequate potassium in the diet.

Rheumatic Fever
- Peaks in school-age children
- Most common cause of acquired heart disease
- Affects connective tissue; most significant complication is mitral valve stenosis.
- Signs and symptoms: a sore throat that appears to be improving (typically follows group A strep infection); then fever develops, along with rash, chorea, and elevated erythrocyte sedimentation rate.

Nursing and Collaborative Management
- Encourage compliance with drug regimens.
  - Penicillin remains the drug of choice.
  - Salicylates are used to control the inflammatory process and reduce fever and discomfort.
  - Prednisone may be indicated in some clients with heart failure.
- Facilitate recovery from the illness.
  - Stress bed rest or at least limited activity during the acute illness.
  - Support secondary prophylaxis.
  - Provide emotional support.

A 2-year-old child's blood work is evaluated by the PN. Considering that the child is prescribed furosemide, captopril, and Lanoxin for congestive heart failure, which value should the PN verify with the laboratory?
A. Hypocalcemia
B. Hypernatremia
C. Low hemoglobin
D. Hypokalemia

HESI Test Question Approach			
Positive?		YES	NO
Key Words			
Rephrase			
Rule Out Choices			
A	B	C	D

A pediatric client is prescribed Lanoxin for a congenital heart defect. The maintenance dosage ordered is 50 mcg/kg/day. The child weighs 10 kg. The prescription requires the Lanoxin to be administered twice daily. How much Lanoxin does the PN prepare to administer to the child with each dose? Round to the nearest hundredth mg/dose. (Fill in the blank.) *250 mcg = 0.25 mg*

The PN reviews the medication record of a 2-month-old and notes that the infant was given a scheduled dose of digoxin with a documented apical pulse of 76 beats/min. What action should the PN take first?
A. Assess the current apical heart rate.
B. Observe for the onset of diarrhea.
C. Complete an adverse occurrence report.
D. Determine the serum potassium level.

HESI Test Question Approach			
Positive?		YES	NO
Key Words			
Rephrase			
Rule Out Choices			
A	B	C	D

Neurological and Muscular Disorders

The PN is caring for a 16-year-old with Down syndrome in a group home. The teenager has a functional age of 5. Which priority nursing action should be included in the plan of care?
A. Monitoring for hearing loss
B. Monitoring intake and output (I & O)
C. Providing a dependable routine
D. Providing a quiet environment

HESI Test Question Approach			
Positive?		YES	NO
Key Words			
Rephrase			
Rule Out Choices			
A	B	C	D

Down Syndrome

- Flat, broad nasal bridge; upward, outward slant of eyes
- Commonly associated problems
  - Cardiac defects
  - Delayed development
  - Respiratory infections
  - Always evaluate functional age
- Feed to back and side of mouth because of tongue thrust.
- Refer family to early intervention program.

NCLEX-PN Exam questions are likely to focus on supporting the child and the parent(s) in order to enable the child to achieve the highest level of functioning.

Cerebral Palsy (CP)

- Chronic, nonprogressive disorder of the motor centers of the brain before, during, or after birth
- Primary disturbances of abnormal muscle tone and coordination
- Diagnosis is made through evaluation of the child. Findings include:
  - Persistent neonatal reflexes after 6 months
  - Spasticity

Nursing and Collaborative Management

- Prevent aspiration with feedings.
- Use of adaptive equipment
- Common drugs for seizures are divalproex, oxycarbamazepine, and lamotrigine.
- Administer diazepam for muscle spasticity; use in older children and adolescents.
- Intrathecal baclofen to decrease spasticity
- Botulinum toxin A decreases muscle pain from spasms.

Spina Bifida Occulta

- No sac is present.
- Suspect if tuft of hair is present at base of spine

Meningocele

- Contains only meninges and spinal fluid
- No nerves are present in spinal sac.

Myelomeningocele

- Sac contains spinal fluid, meninges, and nerves.
- Child has sensory and motor defects.
- Preoperative/postoperative care
  — Monitor urine output.
  — Watch for ↑ ICP.
  — Keep sac free of stool and urine.
  — Measure head circumference every 8 hours and check fontanels.
  — Be alert for signs of latex allergy.

A child with hydrocephalus is 1 day postoperative for revision of a ventriculoatrial shunt. Which finding is most important?
A. Increased blood pressure
B. Increased temperature
C. Increased serum glucose
D. Increased hematocrit

HESI Test Question Approach			
Positive?		YES	NO
Key Words			
Rephrase			
Rule Out Choices			
A	B	C	D

Hydrocephalus

- Abnormal accumulation of cerebrospinal fluid (CSF)
- Symptoms
  — ↑ Intracranial pressure (ICP)
  — ↑ BP
  — ↓ Pulse
  — Changes in level of consciousness
  — Irritability, vomiting
  — Shrill, high-pitched cry in infants

Nursing and Collaborative Management

- Elevate head of bed.
- Use seizure precautions.
- Prepare for shunt placement.
- Assess for shunt malfunctioning.
- Monitor for signs and symptoms of infection.
- Teach parent(s) about shunt replacement.

Seizures or Epilepsy

- Uncontrolled electrical discharges of neurons, more common in children age <2 years
- Seizure types
  — Generalized tonic-clonic (formerly grand mal)
    • Aura precedes seizure
    • Loss of consciousness
    • Tonic phase: stiffness of body
    • Clonic phase: spasms and relaxation
    • Postictal phase: sleepy and disoriented
  — Absence of seizures (formerly petit mal)
    • Momentary loss of consciousness
    • Child appears to be daydreaming.
    • Lasts 5 to 30 seconds

— Myoclonic seizures
  ● Sudden brief contractions of a muscle or group of muscles

Nursing and Collaborative Management

■ Maintain patent airway.
■ Keep side rails up.
■ Pad side rails.
■ Do not use tongue blade.
■ Administer anticonvulsants.
■ Document interventions.
■ Reinforce teaching to family and client about medications.

Anticonvulsants

■ The drug of choice depends on the type of seizure, and the goal is the use of only one drug that will control the seizures with the fewest side effects.
■ Drowsiness, nausea, and loss of appetite are common side effects of many anticonvulsants and may interfere with the child's activities.
■ Careful recording of seizure activity and compliance with the drug regimen are of particular importance.
■ Administer at the same time each day, generally with meals or at bedtime.
  — Phenobarbital
  — Primidone
  — Phenytoin
  — Valproic acid
  — Clonazepam
  — Carbamazepine
  — Ethosuximide
  — Lamotrigine

Bacterial Meningitis

■ Signs and symptoms
  — Older children: signs and symptoms of increased ICP, neck stiffness, plus Kernig's sign, and Brudzinski's sign
  — Infants: classic signs absent; poor feeding, vomiting, irritability, and bulging fontanels
■ Diagnostic procedures include lumbar puncture to obtain sample for laboratory analysis.

Nursing and Collaborative Management

■ Isolate client for at least 24 hours.
■ Administer antibiotics.
■ Obtain baseline VS and perform frequent neurological checks.
■ Assess for ↑ ICP, changes in LOC.
■ Measure head circumference daily.
■ Syndrome of inappropriate antidiuretic hormone (SIADH) occurs frequently.
■ Fluid restrictions may be necessary

Reye's Syndrome

■ Etiology is often but NOT ALWAYS associated with aspirin use and influenza or varicella infection.
■ Rapidly progressing encephalopathy

- Altered hepatic function
- Signs and symptoms: lethargy progressing to coma, vomiting, and hypoglycemia

Nursing and Collaborative Management
- Maintain airway.
- Neurological checks
- Administer mannitol for ICP control.
- Early diagnosis is important to improve client outcome.

Muscular Dystrophy (MD)
Duchenne MD
- Onset between ages 2 and 6 years
- Most severe and most common MD of childhood
- X-linked inherited disease of muscles that leads to atrophy and weakness

Diagnosis
- Muscle biopsy shows degeneration of muscle fibers and replacement with connective tissue and fat.
- Serum creatine phosphokinase (CK) levels are extremely high in early stages, then decrease.

Symptoms
- Delayed walking
- Gower sign
- Frequent falls
- Tiring easily when walking

Nursing and Collaborative Management
- Exercise
- Preventing falls
- Assistive devices for ambulation
- Loss of ambulation: age 8 to 12 years
- Cardiopulmonary complications are most common cause of death.

Renal Disorders in Children

Urinary Tract Infection (UTI)
- More common in girls
- Symptoms
  - Poor food intake
  - Strong-smelling urine
  - Fever
  - Pain with urination

Nursing and Collaborative Management
- Obtain urine culture before starting antibiotics.
- Teach home care.
  - Finish all antibiotics.
  - Avoid bubble baths.
  - Increase intake of fluids.

Acute Glomerulonephritis (AGN)
- Common features
  - Oliguria, hematuria, and proteinuria
  - Edema

— Hypertension
— Circulatory congestion

Nursing Assessment
- Recent strep infection
- Dark, iced tea–colored urine
- Pale, irritable, and/or lethargic

Nursing and Collaborative Management
- Maintenance of fluid balance
- Treatment of hypertension
- Common nursing interventions
  — Frequent vital signs
  — Daily weights
  — Low-sodium
- The client usually recovers without long-term effects.

Nephrotic Syndrome
Nephrotic syndrome is characterized by increased glomerular permeability to protein.

Assessment
- Frothy urine
- Massive proteinuria
- Edema
- Anorexia

Nursing and Collaborative Management
- Reduce excretion of protein.
- Reduce or prevent fluid retention.
- Prevent infections.
- Common interventions
  — Skin care
  — Administer medications
  — No added salt diet
  — Diuretics
  — Prednisone to initiate remission
  — Possible albumin administration
- Discharge teaching
  — Prevent infections
  — Daily weighing
  — Side effects of medications, such as growth retardation from steroids

Acute Renal Failure Management (See Chapter 7.)
A school-age child with nephrotic syndrome is seen at the clinic 2 days after discharge from the hospital. Which assessment is most important after discharge?
A. Pain
B. Capillary refill
C. Urine ketones
D. Daily weight

HESI Test Question Approach			
Positive?		YES	NO
Key Words			
Rephrase			
Rule Out Choices			
A	B	C	D

A 3-week-old baby with pyloric stenosis has severe vomiting. Which sign(s) of dehydration should the PN anticipate the baby presenting? (Select all that apply.)

A.) Sunken fontanel
B. Increased urine output
C.) High serum hematocrit level
D.) Cracked lips
E.) Thirst

HESI Test Question Approach				
Positive?			YES	NO
Key Words				
Rephrase				
Rule Out Choices				
A	B	C	D	E

Gastrointestinal Disorders

Diarrhea

- Worldwide, it is the leading cause of death in children younger than 5 years.
- Rotovirus is one of the leading causes of severe diarrhea in infants and children (immunization with Rotarix).
- Common problem for infants

Symptoms

- Depressed, sunken eyes
- Weight loss
- Decreased urine output

Nursing and Collaborative Management

- Fluid and electrolyte balance
- Rehydration
- Maintenance fluid therapy
- Reintroduction of adequate diet
- Do not give antidiarrheal agents.

Cleft Lip or Cleft Palate

- Malformation of the face or oral cavity
- Initial closure of cleft lip is performed if infant is healthy at or around 3 months of age.
- Closure of cleft palate is performed at about age 1 year.

Nursing and Collaborative Management

- Promote bonding.
- Use Breck or Haberman feeder, slow-flow nipple.
- Maintain airway.
- Do not use straws or spoons.
- Feed only soft foods if child has cleft palate.
- Postoperatively prevent the child from excessive crying, which could cause tension on the suture line, and carefully position (never on the abdomen).

Pyloric Stenosis

- Common in first-born males
- Vomiting becomes projectile around day 14 after birth.
- Dehydration, weight loss, and failure to thrive

Intussusception

- Telescoping of part of the intestine
- Healthy child with a sudden onset of crampy pain, inconsolable crying, and drawing up of knees to chest
- Requires emergency intervention for necrosis and perforation of bowel
- Provide perioperative care for client undergoing repair.

Congenital Aganglionic Megacolon (Hirschsprung's Disease)

- Requires series of surgeries to correct.
- Temporary colostomy is needed, and then at 6 to 12 months of age a rectal pull-through is done.

Hematologic Disorders

- Sickle cell anemia
- Autosomal recessive disorder
- Fetal Hgb does not sickle.
- Hydration to promote hemodilution

Nursing and Collaborative Management

- Crisis marked by fever and pain
- Promote adequate oxygenation.
- Keep well hydrated.
- Do not give supplemental iron.
- Give folic acid orally.

Hemophilia

- X-linked recessive disorder
- Deficiency of missing clotting factors, that is, factor VIII

Nursing and Collaborative Management

- Administer replacement of missing clotting factors.
- Increased risk of bleeding; apply pressure to sites of even minor bleeding.

Metabolic and Endocrine Disorders

Phenylketonuria (PKU)

- Autosomal recessive disorder

A newborn screening for inborn errors of metabolism is drawn 24 hours after birth.

- Strict adherence to low-phenylalanine diet prevents mental disability.
- Special PKU formula
- Avoid meat, dairy, eggs, and foods containing aspartame.
- Eat fruits, juices, cereal, bread, and starches.

Diabetes Mellitus (See Chapter 7.)

Obesity

- Of children age 6 to 11, 19% are categorized as overweight or obese.
- Excess weight and obesity in childhood lead to adult obesity, with increased risks of cardiovascular disease and type 2 diabetes.
- Minorities are disproportionately at risk.

- Parental obesity is the highest predictor of childhood obesity.
- BMI, dietary, and activity assessments should be obtained and evaluated.

Nursing and Collaborative Management for Diabetes
- Consider child's cognitive level and age when planning teaching:
  — Dietary changes
  — Need for exercise
  — Insulin administration
  — Avoid hypoglycemia.
- Continuous follow-up is very important.

Skeletal Disorders

Nursing Assessment
- Visible signs of fractures
- Obtain baseline pulses, color, movement, sensation, temperature, swelling, and pain (5 Ps: pain, pallor, paresthesias, paralysis, and pulses).
- Report any changes immediately.

Traction
Traction is used for fractures that are not easily reducible by casting and for presurgical stabilization of fracture.
- Buck's traction
  — For knee immobilization
- Russell's traction
  — For fracture of femur or lower leg
- 90°/90° traction
  — Pinned for desired line of pull and flexion at hip and knee of 90°

Nursing and Collaborative Management
- Monitor neurovascular status (5 Ps).
- Provide appropriate toys.
- Teach cast care to family.
  — Prevent soiling of cast with careful diapering.

Congenital Dislocated Hip
Assessment
- Positive Ortolani's sign
- Unequal fold of skin on buttocks
- Limited abduction of hip
- Apply Pavlik harness; worn 24 hr/day up to 6 months.
- Treated by surgical correction after 6 months of closed reduction and hip spica cast if Pavlik harness is not effective.

Nursing and Collaborative Management
- Postoperative interventions
- Hip spica cast care

Scoliosis
- S-shaped curvature of the spine
- Most common nontraumatic skeletal condition in children
- Milwaukee brace
- Affects both genders at any age, but is most commonly seen in adolescents.

Juvenile Idiopathic Arthritis (JIA)

- Most common arthritic condition of childhood
- Inflammatory diseases involving the joints, connective tissues, and viscera
- Exact cause is unknown, but infections and autoimmune response have been implicated.
- Therapy consists of administration of medications (e.g., NSAIDs, methotrexate, biologic agents, interleukin or aspirin); exercise; heat application; and support of joints.

A 12-year-old child is admitted with sickle cell crisis. She is anemic and has painful joints and a fever of 101°F. Which priority intervention should the PN include in the plan of care for this child?
A. Maintain oral fluids for hydration.
B. Apply cold packs to painful joints.
C. Administer aspirin daily for pain and fever.
D. Perform range of motion to decrease joint pain.

HESI Test Question Approach		
Positive?	YES	NO
Key Words		
Rephrase		
Rule Out Choices		
A	B	C	D

The PN walks into a hospital room and observes a teenage client experiencing a tonic-clonic seizure. Which intervention should the nurse provide first?
A. Restrain the client to protect against injury.
B. Flex the neck to ensure stabilization.
C. Use a tongue blade to open the airway.
D. Turn the client on side to aid ventilation.

HESI Test Question Approach		
Positive?	YES	NO
Key Words		
Rephrase		
Rule Out Choices		
A	B	C	D

The healthcare provider prescribes the anticonvulsant phenytoin for an adolescent with a seizure disorder. The nurse should instruct the client to notify the healthcare provider if which condition develops?
A. Dry mouth
B. Dizziness
C. Sore throat
D. Gingival hyperplasia

HESI Test Question Approach		
Positive?	YES	NO
Key Words		
Rephrase		
Rule Out Choices		
A	B	C	D

10 Newborn Health Nursing

A client who has reached 36 weeks' gestation is placed in the lithotomy position. She suddenly complains of feeling breathless and lightheaded, and she shows marked pallor. What action should the nurse take first?

A. Turn the client to a lateral position.
B. Place the client in the Trendelenburg position.
C. Obtain vital signs and a pulse oximetry reading.
D. Initiate distraction techniques.

HESI Test Question Approach			
Positive?		YES	NO
Key Words			
Rephrase			
Rule Out Choices			
A	B	C	D

Pregnancy: Key Assessments

- Assess for violence
  - Battering and emotional or physical abuse can begin with pregnancy.
  - In private away from partner, assess for abuse.
  - The nurse needs to know about local resources and how to determine client's safety.
- Gravidity and parity counts pregnancies, not offspring.
  - Gravida is the number of times a female has been pregnant, regardless of outcome.
  - Para is the number of deliveries (not children) that occurred after 20 weeks' gestation.
    - Multiple births count as one.
    - Loss of pregnancy before 20 weeks counted as abortion, but add one to gravidity.
    - Fetal demise after 20 weeks added to parity.
- The acronym *GTPAL* represents obstetric history.
  G: Gravidity (the number of pregnancies)
  T: Term pregnancies after 37 weeks
  P: Preterm pregnancies prior to 37 weeks
  A: Abortions (elective or spontaneous), a loss prior to 20 weeks
  L: Living children
- Gestation
  - Naegele's rule: Count back 3 months from date of last normal menstrual period; add 1 year and 7 days.
    - *Example:* If the last menstrual period was May 2, 2017, the EDB would be February 9, 2018.
- Fundal height
  - 12 to 13 weeks: Fundus rises out of symphysis.
  - 20 weeks: Fundus is at the umbilicus.
  - 24 to about 36 weeks: Fundal height (in centimeters) from the symphysis is equal to the number of weeks of gestation if this is a single pregnancy.

- Weight gain: Optimal weight gain depends on maternal and fetal factors.
  — In first trimester, average total weight gain is 1 to 2 kg.
  — Approximately 0.5 kg per week for a woman of normal weight during second and third trimesters
- Maternal psychological changes
  — Ambivalence occurs early in pregnancy, even with a planned pregnancy.
  — Acceptance occurs with the woman's readiness for the experience and identification with the motherhood role. Prolonged nonacceptance of the pregnancy is a warning sign but not directly related to nonacceptance of the child.
  — Emotional lability: rapid, unpredictable changes in mood

A client's suspected pregnancy is confirmed. The client tells the PN that she has had previous pregnancies: She delivered a single child at 39 weeks, twins at 34 weeks, and a single child at 35 weeks. Using the GTPAL notation system, how should the PN record the client's gravidity and parity?
A. 3-0-3-0-3
B. 3-1-1-1-3
C. 4-1-2-0-4
D. 4-2-1-0-3

HESI Test Question Approach			
Positive?		YES	NO
Key Words			
Rephrase			
Rule Out Choices			
A	B	C	D

External fetal monitoring is noninvasive and is performed with a Toco transducer for uterine activity and Doppler ultrasonic transducer for FHR

Internal fetal monitoring is invasive; the membranes must be ruptured, and an electrode must be attached to the presenting part of the fetus to monitor fetal heart rate.

Intrauterine catheter is used to monitor for contractions

Nursing and Collaborative Care During Labor
- Assessment
  — Cultural factors influence the response to labor and coping.
  — Emotional response: support and coping
  — Pain and discomfort: medications and nonpharmacological measures
  — Response to medications: epidural and Pitocin
  — Maternal vital signs
  — Fetal heart rate pattern
  — Uterine activity
  — Fetal position: Leopold's maneuvers and vaginal exam
- Assessment of labor progression: dilatation, effacement, and descent
  — Status of the membranes: prevent and detect infection

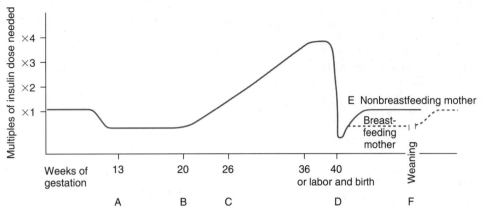

Fig. 10-1 Changing insulin needs during pregnancy. A is the first trimester: Insulin need is reduced because of increased insulin production by pancreas and increased peripheral sensitivity to insulin; nausea, vomiting, and decreased food intake by mother and glucose transfer to embryo or fetus contribute to hypoglycemia. B is the second trimester: Insulin needs begin to increase as placental hormones, cortisol, and insulinase act as insulin antagonists, decreasing insulin's effectiveness. C is third trimester: Insulin needs may double or even quadruple but usually level off after 36 weeks of gestation. D is day of birth: Maternal insulin requirements decrease drastically to approach prepregnancy levels. E: Breastfeeding mother maintains lower insulin requirements, as much as 25% less than those of prepregnancy; insulin needs of nonbreastfeeding mother return to prepregnancy levels in 7 to 10 days. F: Weaning of breastfeeding infant causes mother's insulin needs to return to prepregnancy levels. (Lowdermilk, D., Perry, S., Cashion, K., Alden, K.R. (2012). *Maternity and women's health care* (10th ed.). St. Louis: Mosby.)

— Nutrient and fluid intake: hydration and bladder status, need for catheterization, and IV therapy
— Bowel elimination
— Labs and diagnostic tests
— Assess for signs of complications: infection, pregnancy-induced hypertension (PIH), bleeding, prolapsed cord, and fetal distress.
— Ambulation and positioning: upright, sitting, and squatting best

Types of Regional Blocks Used to Manage Labor Discomfort

- Pudendal block
  — Given for episiotomy
  — Has no effect on pain of uterine contractions.
- Peridural (epidural or caudal) block
  — Given in first or second stage
  — Single dose or given continuously
  — May prolong second stage.
  — Fluid bolus to prevent hypotension
  — Increases risk for urinary retention and need for catheterization.
- Intradural (subarachnoid, spinal)
  — Given in second stage
  — Rapid onset
  — Client must remain flat for 6 to 8 hours after delivery.

Postpartum Care

Postpartum Maternal Physical Assessment Summary

- Memory tool BUBBLE HA

- Breasts: Assess consistency (soft, firm, filling, or engorged), nipples (intact, soreness, flat, everted, or inverted), and masses
- Uterus: Fundal involution. Immediately after delivery the fundus is several centimeters below the umbilicus; within 12 hours it rises to the umbilicus and descends 1 cm (a fingerbreadth) per day for 9 to 10 days, putting it below the symphysis pubis; it should be in the midline and firm.
- Bladder: Measure output; assess for distention or retention.
- Bowel: Assess for distention, passing flatus, and bowel sounds.
- Lochia: Endometrial sloughing from rubra to serosa to alba; assess color, odor, and volume.
- Leg: Assess for signs of thrombosis.
- Episiotomy: Assess episiotomy or laceration repair for intactness, hematoma, edema, bruising, redness, and drainage.
- Hemorrhoids: Treat with sitz bath, Tucks pads, and ointments
- Attachment: Assess maternal–infant interaction for bonding behaviors.

Teaching Points

Priority focus is on signs of physical and psychoemotional symptoms of potential problems for mother and infant and how to obtain help.

- Change pads as needed and with voiding and defecation. Wipe front to back.
- Practice good handwashing technique.
- Ice packs, sitz baths, peri bottle lavage, and topical anesthetic spray and pads
- Breastfeeding instructions
- Balanced diet and adequate fluid intake
- Rest/nap when baby sleeps
- Contraceptive use

Rh₀(D) Immune Globulin (RhoGAM) (WinRho®, Given to Rh-Negative Women with Possible Exposure to Rh-Positive Blood)

- Should have negative indirect Coombs test.
- Given IM within 72 hours after delivery
- Must be checked by two nurses (blood product).

Rubella Vaccine

- Given subcutaneously to nonimmune client before discharge from hospital
- May breastfeed.
- Do not give if client or family member is immunocompromised.
- Avoid pregnancy for 2 to 3 months (reinforce contraception).

A client who is 72 hours post cesarean section is preparing to go home. She complains to the PN that she can't get the baby's diaper on right. Which action should the nurse take?

A. Demonstrate how to diaper the baby correctly.

B. Observe the client diapering the baby while offering praise and hints.

C. Call the social worker for long-term follow-up.

D. Reassure the client that she knows how to take care of her baby.

<table>
<tr><td colspan="3">HESI Test Question Approach</td></tr>
<tr><td>Positive?</td><td>YES</td><td>NO</td></tr>
<tr><td>Key Words</td><td></td><td></td></tr>
<tr><td></td><td></td><td></td></tr>
<tr><td></td><td></td><td></td></tr>
<tr><td>Rephrase</td><td></td><td></td></tr>
<tr><td></td><td></td><td></td></tr>
<tr><td></td><td></td><td></td></tr>
<tr><td colspan="3">Rule Out Choices</td></tr>
<tr><td>A</td><td>B</td><td>C   D</td></tr>
</table>

Complications

Chronic Hypertension

- Hypertension and/or proteinuria in pregnant woman: chronic hypertension occurs before 20 weeks of gestation; persistent hypertension occurs 12 weeks postpartum.

Superimposed Preeclampsia or Eclampsia

- Development of preeclampsia or eclampsia in a woman with chronic hypertension before 20 weeks of gestation

Preeclampsia/Eclampsia

Preeclampsia Symptoms

- BP
  - *Mild:* 30 mm Hg systolic and/or 15 mm Hg diastolic over baseline
  - *Severe:* same (some sources say 160/110 mm Hg × 2 or more readings)
- Protein
  - Mild: >1+
  - Severe: 3+ to 4+
- Edema
  - *Mild:* eyes, face, fingers
  - *Severe:* generalized edema
- Deep tendon reflexes (DTRs)
  - *Mild:* may be normal
  - *Severe:* 3+ or more and clonus
- Central nervous system (CNS) symptoms
  - *Mild:* headache, irritability
  - *Severe:* severe headache, visual disturbances
- Other
  - Weight gain >2 lb/week
  - Oliguria (<100 mL/4 hr), epigastric pain related to liver enlargement
  - Elevated serum creatinine, thrombocytopenia, and marked SGOT elevation

Nursing and Collaborative Management

Preeclampsia

- Minimize stimulation in room.
- Explain procedures.

- Maintain IV (16- to 18-g venocatheter).
- Monitor BP every 15 to 30 minutes.
- Monitor urine for protein every hour.
- Healthcare provider may prescribe magnesium sulfate.

Nursing and Collaborative Management

Eclampsia (Seizures)
- Stay with client.
- Turn client to side.
- Do not attempt to force objects into client's mouth.
- Administer O_2 and have suction available.

Gestational Diabetes

Screening
- Recommendations for glucose screening for all pregnant women:
  — 1-hour glucose screening between 24 and 26 weeks
  — Goal is strict blood glucose control.
  — Generally, Glyburide or insulin is used during pregnancy. Insulin does not cross the placenta; Glyburide minimally crosses it.

A client who has gestational diabetes asks the PN to explain why her baby is at risk for macrosomia. Which explanation should the nurse offer?
A. The placenta receives decreased maternal blood flow during pregnancy because of vascular constriction.
B. The fetus secretes insulin in response to maternal hyperglycemia, causing weight gain and growth.
C. Infants of diabetic mothers are postmature, which allows the fetus extra time to grow.
D. Rapid fetal growth contributes to congenital anomalies, which are more common in infants of diabetic mothers.

HESI Test Question Approach		
Positive?	YES	NO
Key Words		
Rephrase		
Rule Out Choices		
A	B	C	D

Preterm Labor (PTL)

Signs and Symptoms
- More than five contractions per hour; menstrual-like cramps.
- Low, dull backache
- Pelvic pressure
- Increase/change in vaginal discharge
- Leaking or gush of amniotic fluid

Tocolytics and Their Administration
A number of medications can be used to stop uterine contractions:
  - Low K^+, hyperglycemia
  — Nursing interventions
    - Maternal ECG and lab tests
    - Cardiac and fetal monitoring
    - VS every 15 min
  — Antidote
    - Propranolol (Inderal)

- Terbutaline (Brethine)
  - — Side effects
    - Nervousness, tremulousness
    - Headache
    - Nausea/vomiting, diarrhea, epigastric pain
  - — Adverse effects
    - Tachycardia
    - Chest pain with pulmonary edema
    - Low K^+, hyperglycemia
  - — Nursing interventions
    - Hold and notify HCP if maternal pulse >130 beats/min or FHR >180 beats/min.
    - Monitor I & O.
    - Check weight daily.
  - — Antidote
    - Propranolol (Inderal)
- Magnesium sulfate
  - — Side effects
    - CNS depression
    - Slowed respirations
    - Decreased DTRs
  - — Adverse effects
    - Decreased urine output
    - Pulmonary edema
  - — Nursing interventions
    - Hold if respirations are <12 breaths/min, urine output <100 mL/4 hr, and absent DTRs.
    - Monitor serum magnesium levels: Therapeutic range is between 4 and 7.5 mEq/L or 5 to 8 mg/dL.
  - — Antidote
    - Calcium gluconate
- Other drugs used to reduce contractions:
  - — Indomethacin
  - — Naproxen
  - — Nifedipine (Procardia)

A client at 15 weeks' gestation is admitted for an inevitable abortion. Thirty minutes after her return from surgery, her vital signs are stable. Which nursing intervention has the highest priority?

A. Ask the client whether she would like to talk about losing her baby.

B. Place cold cabbage leaves on the client's breasts to reduce breast engorgement.

C. Send a referral to the grief counselor for at-home follow-up.

D. Confirm the client's Rh and Coombs status and administer RhoGAM if indicated.

HESI Test Question Approach			
Positive?		YES	NO
Key Words			
Rephrase			
Rule Out Choices			
A	B	C	D

Spontaneous Abortion

Assessment

- Vaginal bleeding at week 20 of gestation or earlier
- Uterine cramping, backache, and pelvic pressure
- May have symptoms of shock
- Assess client's and family members' emotional status, needs, and support.

Nursing and Collaborative Management

- Monitor VS, LOC, and amount of bleeding.
- Prepare client to receive IV fluids and/or blood.
- If client is Rh negative, administer RhoGAM.

Incompetent Cervix

- Recurrent premature dilation of the cervix and is defined as passive and painless dilation of the cervix during the second trimester.
- Conservative management
  — Bed rest
  — Hydration
  — Tocolysis (inhibition of uterine contractions)
- Cervical cerclage may be performed.
  — Postoperative nursing care: Monitor uterine activity, bleeding, rupture of membranes, and signs of infection.
- Administer tocolytics.
- Discharge teaching: Teach to report signs of labor, bleeding, and infection; decrease activity to x 1 week and pelvic rest.

Ectopic Pregnancy

Assessment

- Missed period, but early signs of pregnancy absent
- Positive result on pregnancy test
- Rupture
  — Sharp, unilateral pelvic pain
  — Vaginal bleeding
  — Referred shoulder pain
  — Syncope can lead to shock

Nursing and Collaborative Management

- Monitor client's hemodynamic status.
- Prepare client for surgery and administration of IV fluids, including blood.

Abruptio Placentae and Placenta Previa

Abruptio Placentae

- Concealed or overt bleeding
- Uterine tone ranges from tense without relaxation to tense and board-like.
- Persistently painful
- Abnormal fetal heart rate (complete abruption = absent FHR)

Placenta Previa

- Bright red vaginal bleeding
- Soft uterine tone
- Painless

- FHR is normal unless bleeding is severe and mother becomes hypovolemic.

Disseminated Intravascular Coagulation (DIC)
- Risk factors for DIC in pregnancy
  - Fetal demise
  - Infection and/or sepsis
  - Pregnancy-induced hypertension (preeclampsia)
  - Abruptio placentae

Dystocia
Dystocia is a difficult birth that occurs because of problems involving one or more of the 5 Ps (powers, passage, passenger, psyche, and position). Examples include lack of progress in cervical dilation, delay in fetal descent, or a change in the characteristics of uterine contraction.

Postpartum Complications
- Hemorrhage
  - Assess fundal location and consistency.
  - Assess vaginal bleeding: Saturating one pad per hour = hemorrhage.
  - Monitor for signs of shock.
  - Assess for bladder distention, can prevent involution and lead to hemorrhage.
- Venous thromboembolism is related to venous stasis and hypercoagulability.
  - Can result in superficial venous thrombosis, DVT, or pulmonary embolism
  - Assess legs for pain, tenderness, swelling (Homan's sign not reliable).
  - Treated with bed rest, anticoagulants, leg elevation, and analgesia

Postpartum Infections
- Perineal infections
- Endometritis
- Parametritis
- Peritonitis
- Mastitis
- Deep vein thrombosis
- Cystitis
- Pyelonephritis
- HIV, hepatitis, and other STIs

Which nursing action has the highest priority for an infant immediately after birth?
A. Place the infant's head in the sniffing position and give oxygen via face mask.
B. Perform a bedside glucose test and feed the infant glucose water as needed.
C. Assess the heart rate and perform chest compressions if the rate is below 60 beats/min.
D. Dry the infant and place him or her under a radiant warmer or skin to skin with the mother.

HESI Test Question Approach			
Positive?		**YES**	**NO**
Key Words			
Rephrase			
Rule Out Choices			
A	**B**	**C**	**D**

Newborn Parameters (Approximate)

- Length: 18 to 22 inches
- Weight: 5.5 to 9.5 lb
- Head circumference: 13.2 to 14 inches
- Sutures palpable with fontanels
- Fontanel closure
  — Anterior: by 18 months
  — Posterior: 6 to 8 weeks
- Umbilical cord should have three vessels: two arteries and one vein.
- Extremities should be flexed.
- Major gluteal folds should be even.
- Creases should be present on soles of feet.
- Ortolani's sign and Barlow's sign should be assessed for developmental dysplasia of the hip.
- Pulses should be palpable (radial, brachial, and femoral).

Nursing and Collaborative Management

- Keep newborn warm.
- Suction airway as needed.
- Observe for respiratory distress.
- Normal or physiological jaundice appears after the first 24 hours in full-term newborns.
- Pathological jaundice occurs before this time and may indicate early hemolysis of red blood cells.
- Assess hemoglobin and hematocrit (H & H) and blood glucose levels.
- Weigh daily.
- Monitor intake and output; weigh diapers if necessary (1 g = 1 mL of urine).
- Monitor temperature.
- Observe for cracks in skin.
- Administer eye medication within 1 hour after birth.
- Provide cord care.
- Provide circumcision care. Teach client how to care for circumcision site.
- Supine position ("Back to sleep") to prevent SIDs.
- Observe for normal stool and passage of meconium.
- Test newborn's reflexes.

Ages at Which Infant Reflexes Disappear

- Sucking or rooting: 3 to 4 months
- Moro: 3 to 4 months
- Tonic neck or fencing: 3 to 4 months
- Babinski's sign: 1 year to 18 months
- Palmar-plantar grasp: 8 months
- Stepping or walking: 3 to 4 months

Major Newborn Complications

Hypoglycemia

- Assess for risk factors in maternal history (infant of diabetic mother) and environmental factors (cold stress).
- In general, blood glucose levels <40 mg/dL are considered abnormal and warrant investigation and intervention.

- Infant is fed formula or breastfed as soon as the repeat (usually) sample is obtained to prevent a further drop in blood glucose.
- Administer intravenous glucose infusions per HCP prescription for infants with symptomatic hypoglycemia or those too ill to be fed orally safely.
- Reduce adverse environmental factors (e.g., excessive handling, and cold stress).

Respiratory Distress Syndrome
- Causes inability to produce surfactant
- Results in hypoxia and acidosis

Meconium Aspiration Syndrome
- Fetal distress increases intestinal peristalsis.
- Releases meconium into the amniotic fluid.

Retinopathy of Prematurity
- Damage to retinal vessels is caused by prolonged use of oxygen (>30 days).
- Infants receiving oxygen therapy to be examined by ophthalmologist.

Hyperbilirubinemia
- Elevated serum levels: >12 mg/dL
- Crucial to prevent kernicterus, which results in permanent neurological damage
- Jaundice starts at head, spreads to chest, abdomen, arms, legs, hands, and feet.
- Treated with phototherapy, use of fluorescent lights to reduce serum bilirubin levels
  — Possible adverse effects: eye damage, dehydration, and sensory deprivation
  — Expose as much of the skin as possible, but cover genital area.
  — Cover eyes with eye shields.
  — Monitor skin temperature closely.
  — Increase fluids to compensate for water loss.
  — Expect loose, green stools and green urine.
  — Monitor newborn's skin color.
  — Reposition every 2 hours.
  — Provide stimulation.
  — After treatment, continue monitoring for signs of rebound hyperbilirubinemia.

Erythroblastosis Fetalis
- Results from Rh negative (RH−) mother exposed to Rh positive (Rh+) blood and develops antibodies that are passed to the fetus, destroying fetal red blood cells
- Characterized by hemolytic anemia or hyperbilirubinemia
- Administer $Rh_0(D)$ immune globulin to RH− mother to prevent development of maternal antibodies.
- Treatment of newborn includes phototherapy and exchange transfusion.

CBRN

Sepsis

- Presence of bacteria in the blood
- Prevention: antibiotics in labor for positive group B streptococci (GBS) test
- Assess for maternal, intrapartum, and neonatal risk factors.
- Early signs are nonspecific and include lethargy, poor feeding, poor weight gain, temperature instability, and irritability.

TORCH Infections

TORCH group of infections includes:

T: Toxoplasmosis

O: Other infections (e.g., gonorrhea, syphilis, varicella, hepatitis B, HIV, or human parvovirus B19)

R: Rubella

C: Cytomegalovirus

H: Herpes simplex virus

Substance Abuse

- Effects on fetus vary according to substance.
- Narcotics cause passive addiction—neonatal abstinence syndrome.
- Cocaine is classified as a narcotic but not an opioid; it causes vasoconstriction, preterm birth, poor growth, and neurological problems.

Fetal Alcohol Syndrome

- Caused by maternal alcohol use during pregnancy
- Associated with neurological problems, IQ deficit, and attention deficit hyperactivity disorder
- Craniofacial features include microcephaly, small eyes or short palpebral fissures, a thin upper lip, a flat midface, and an indistinct philtrum.
- Treatment of drug-exposed newborns focuses on reduction of external stimuli, supportive treatment of symptoms, and sedation.

Newborn of Mother with HIV

- Monitor antibodies closely throughout pregnancy.
- Testing and treatment in pregnancy greatly reduce risk of transmission to fetus.

Infant of Diabetic Mother (IDM)

- Infant born to mother with insulin-dependent or gestational diabetes
- Newborn may have hypoglycemia, hypocalcemia, hypomagnesemia, polycythemia, hyperbilirubinemia, cardiomyopathy, respiratory distress syndrome (RDS), birth trauma, and congenital anomalies.

A pregnant client tells the PN that she smokes only a few cigarettes a day. What information should the nurse provide the client about the effects of smoking during pregnancy?

A. Smoking causes vasoconstriction and reduces placental perfusion.
B. Smoking reduces the lecithin-sphingomyelin (L:S) ratio, contributing to lung immaturity.
C. Smoking causes vasodilation and fluid overload for the fetus.
D. Smoking during pregnancy places the fetus at risk for lung cancer.

HESI Test Question Approach			
Positive?		YES	NO
Key Words			
Rephrase			
Rule Out Choices			
A	B	C	D

11 Mental Health Nursing

An adult client is admitted to the inpatient mental health unit for severe depression. Although the client has agreed to electroconvulsive therapy (ECT), the client's partner states, "I've heard that that ECT destroys neurons and that memory loss is significant." Which response by the practical nurse is most helpful?

A. I'll contact the nursing supervisor for you.
B. Talking with the ECT staff may help you feel more comfortable.
C. I think you should show support for your partner.
D. Perhaps you and I can discuss your concerns about ECT.

HESI Test Question Approach			
Positive?		**YES**	**NO**
Key Words			
Rephrase			
Rule Out Choices			
A	**B**	**C**	**D**

Therapeutic Communication

- Both nonverbal and verbal expression. Nonverbal communication may be most important.
- Goal directed: Assist client with ADLs or discuss problem.
- Appropriate, effective, and flexible; includes feedback loop.

Important Definitions

Mental health: Successful adjustment to changing internal and external environments; achieving mental health (and sustaining it) is a lifelong process.

The nurse and client relationship is a therapeutic relationship in which the nurse's goal is to help the client in developing problem-solving skills to facilitate activities of daily living and to promote self-care and independence when appropriate.

Mental illness is a loss of the ability to respond to the environment (i.e., successfully adjust to changes) in accord with oneself and society.

Privacy and confidentiality are the client's reasonable expectations that information revealed to the nurse will be disclosed to other members of the interprofessional team but not to the client's family or friends. The nurse is responsible for notifying the treatment team immediately if the client has thoughts of harming self or others.

A female client who has just learned that she has breast cancer tells her family that the biopsy result was negative. What action should the nurse take?

A. Remind the client that the result was positive.
B. Ask the client to restate what the healthcare provider told her.
C. Talk to the family about the client's need for family support.
D. Encourage the client to talk to the nurse about her fears.

HESI Test Question Approach			
Positive?		**YES**	**NO**
Key Words			
Rephrase			
Rule Out Choices			
A	**B**	**C**	**D**

Coping and Defense Mechanisms

- Efforts to reduce anxiety
- Can be constructive or destructive
- *Coping* is related to problem-solving
- *Defense* is related to protecting oneself

Therapeutic Treatment Modalities

Milieu therapy: physical and social environment in which client is receiving treatment

Interpersonal psychotherapy: use of a therapeutic relationship to modify client's feelings, attitudes, and behaviors

Behavior therapy: can take many forms; used to change client's behaviors.

Cognitive therapy: a directive, time-limited approach

Electroconvulsive therapy (ECT): use of electrically induced seizures to treat severely depressed individuals who fail to respond to antidepressant medications and therapy

Group Therapy

- Involves a therapist and 5 to 8 members
- Interactions among group members provide feedback and support for group and individual goals

Group Therapy Types

- Interpersonal group therapy
- Self-help or support groups
- Family therapy
  — Family member with the presenting symptoms indicates presence of problems in the entire family.
- Change in one family member brings about changes in the others.

The PN and mental health technician are assigned a group of mental health clients to lead in bingo, a social activity. During the game, a client begins to complain of shortness of breath and dizziness. Which intervention should the nurse provide first?

A. Ask a technician to escort the client back to the unit.
B. Ask the client to describe current feelings.
C. Lead the client to a quiet area.
D. Request an additional staff member.

HESI Test Question Approach			
Positive?		**YES**	**NO**
Key Words			
Rephrase			
Rule Out Choices			
A	**B**	**C**	**D**

Anxiety

- A normal, subjective experience that includes feelings of apprehension, uneasiness, uncertainty, or dread

Severe stress may create levels of anxiety leading to depression, helplessness, and hopelessness that can end in panic.

Types of Anxiety

- *Mild:* tension of everyday life
- *Moderate*: immediate concerns
- *Severe:* feeling that something bad is about to happen
- *Panic:* terror and sense of impending doom

Anxiety Disorders

- *Generalized anxiety disorder:* unrealistic anxiety about everyday worries occurring over a long time period
- *Panic disorder:* produces sudden feeling of intense apprehension, fear, or worry.
- *Phobia:* irrational fear of an object, activity, or situation
  - Client may recognize fear as unreasonable.
  - Associated with panic-level anxiety
  - Defense mechanisms include repression and displacement (i.e., claustrophobia).

Nursing and Collaborative Management

- Reduce stimuli in environment.
- Provide calm, quiet environment.
- Administer antianxiety medications as prescribed.
- Administer SSRIs and tricyclic antidepressants as prescribed.

Antianxiety (Anxiolytic) Medications

Benzodiazepines are usually prescribed for a brief period.

- Benzodiazepines depress the CNS; they have anxiety-reducing (anxiolytic), sedative-hypnotic, muscle-relaxing, and anticonvulsant actions.
- Flumazenil (Romazicon), a benzodiazepine antagonist administered IV, reverses benzodiazepine intoxication in 5 minutes.

Somatic Symptom Disorders
- Persistent worry or complaints regarding physical illness without physical findings
- Types of somatoform disorders
  — Conversion disorder
  — Hypochondriasis
  — Somatization disorders
- Treatment: cognitive-behavioral therapy

The PN is reinforcing education to a client for coping with anxiety when the client is seen washing hands compulsively. What action should the PN take next?
A. Discuss alternatives to handwashing while the client continues washing hands.
B. Ask client to stop washing hands immediately.
C. Allow client to finish washing hands before teaching.
D. Ask client what triggered the handwashing.

HESI Test Question Approach		
Positive?	YES	NO
Key Words		
Rephrase		
Rule Out Choices		

A	B	C	D

Crisis Intervention
- A crisis results from experiencing a significant traumatic event or situation that the client cannot remedy by the use of the client's available coping strategies.
- Crises are time-limited events that are usually resolved within 6 weeks.
- Types of crises
  — Maturational (midlife crisis)
  — Situational (sudden death of loved one)
  — Adventitious (disaster associated with a tornado)
- Goal is to return client to precrisis level of functioning.

Nursing and Collaborative Management
- Evaluate for suicidal or homicidal thoughts or plans or other indications for hospitalization.
- Identify the client's usual coping mechanisms.
- Evaluate the client's perception of the present situation.
- Ascertain religious or cultural beliefs that need to be considered when developing interventions.
- Determine how this crisis affects the client's life. For example, can the client work?
- Mobilize efforts to meet the need for safety and decrease anxiety.
- Involve the client in identifying realistic, acceptable interventions.

Traumatic and Stressor–Related Disorders

- Includes severe anxiety that occurs as result of direct or indirect exposure to a traumatic event (rape, war, and terror) that may also include persistent reexperiencing of the precipitating trauma.

Symptoms: intrusive thoughts, negative mood, or hyperarousal

PTSD's Four Symptom Clusters
- Avoidance reminders of the event
- Continuing negative changes in mood and thoughts
- Recurring negative emotional states
- Reckless behavior such as suicidal ideation, substance abuse, or increasing irritable or aggressive behavior

Other Stressor-Related Disorders
- Anxiety displayed in symptoms
  - Intrusive thoughts
  - Nightmares
  - Emotional detachment
  - Flashbacks
- Responses include shock, anger, denial or panic, and/or self-destructive behavior (e.g., substance abuse or suicidal ideation).
- Reactions may be triggered by visible reminders of the trauma (e.g. physical disabilities).

Nursing and Collaborative Management
- Assess suicidal risk.
- Actively listen to stories of the experiences that occurred around the traumatic event.
- Encourage participation in group therapy with others who have experienced related traumatic events.
- Assist client to solve problems by identify previous successful coping skills.
- Administer prescribed medication to decrease anxiety, provide rest, and manage behavior.

Personality Disorder Types

- Antisocial
- Borderline
- Obsessive-compulsive

Antisocial personality disorder
- Has aggressive acting-out behavior patterns
- No remorse for actions or behavior
- Manipulative in meeting own needs
- Humiliating, belligerent, and disparaging actions toward others
- Often socially gracious to achieve own ends
- Example: prisoners who seduce guards to assist in escapes

Obsessive-compulsive disorder
- Obsessions: persistently intrusive thoughts
- Compulsions: repetitive behaviors designed to divert unacceptable thought and reduce anxiety (i.e., hoarding disorder)

Borderline personality disorder
- Inflexible, maladaptive behavior patterns
- Client in touch with reality
- Client lacks insight into his or her behavior.
- Forms of acting out
  - Yelling and swearing
  - Cutting own skin
  - Manipulation
  - Substance abuse
  - Promiscuous sexual behavior
  - Suicide attempts

Nursing and Collaborative Management
- Multiple psychotherapies are required to aid behavior change and promote satisfactory relationships.
- Be alert to splitting and suicidal ideation.
- Pharmacological intervention comprises a broad range, including antianxiety agents, antidepressants, and antipsychotic drugs.

A female client who is diagnosed with borderline personality disorder returns after a weekend pass with lacerations to both wrists. The client vigorously complains to the nurse during the dressing change. The PN's response should be:
A. Distant
B. Attentive
C. Matter of fact
D. Compassionate

HESI Test Question Approach			
Positive?		**YES**	**NO**
Key Words			
Rephrase			
Rule Out Choices			
A	**B**	**C**	**D**

Eating Disorders

Compulsive Overeating
- Binge-like overeating without purging
- Caused by lack of control over food consumption

Anorexia Nervosa
- Onset often associated with stressful event
- Client experiences altered body image.
- Death can occur from starvation, suicide, cardiomyopathies, or electrolyte imbalance.

Bulimia Nervosa
- Binge-purge syndrome: eating binges followed by purging behaviors

A client with bulimia is admitted to the mental health unit. What intervention is most important for the PN to include in the initial treatment plan?
A. Observe the client after meals for vomiting.
B. Assess daily weight and vital signs.
C. Monitor serum potassium and calcium levels.
D. Provide a structured environment at mealtimes.

HESI Test Question Approach			
Positive?		**YES**	**NO**
Key Words			
Rephrase			
Rule Out Choices			
A	**B**	**C**	**D**

Depressive Disorders

Depression

- Characterized by feelings of hopelessness and low self-esteem, as well as a tendency to take the blame for every negative event
- 25% of those with depression have suicidal ideation,
- Behavior therapy, cognitive behavioral therapy, and interpersonal psychotherapy all reduce symptoms of depression and maintain their effects well after treatment has ended.
- Antidepressant medication therapy
  — Cyclic antidepressants (e.g., TCAs)
  — SSRIs and SNRIs
  — Atypical antidepressants

Suicide

- Suicide threat is a warning, direct or indirect, verbal or nonverbal, that a person is planning to take his or her own life.
- The person may give away prized possessions, make a will or funeral arrangements, or withdraw from friendships and social activities.
- Assessment includes whether the person has made a specific plan and whether the means to carry out the plan are available.
- Treatment: The highest priority is to protect the client from inflicting harm, being vigilant, supervise medication administration, implementing strategies to increase self-esteem, and increase social support.

Bipolar Disorders

- Characterized by episodes of mania and depression between which the client has periods of normal mood and activity
- Treatment: Lithium carbonate, the medication of choice, can be toxic and requires regular monitoring of serum lithium levels.
  — Other medications
    • Divalproex (Valproate)
    • Olanzapine (Zyprexa)
    • Carbamazepine (Tegretol)

Nursing and Collaborative Management
High-Alert Antidepressant Use

- *Serotonin syndrome:* Hyperthermia rigidity, cognitive impairments, and autonomic symptoms. Potentially fatal and may occur at any time during therapy with serotonin reuptake inhibitor medication (SSRIs) combined with monamine oxidase inhibitors (MAOIs). Treatment is symptomatic with propranolol, cooling blankets, chlorpromazine for hyperthermia, diazepam for muscle rigidity or rigors.
- *Antidepressant apathy:* Some clients lose interest in life and the events around them.
- *Antidepressant withdrawal syndrome:* Abrupt cessation of antidepressants engenders withdrawal symptoms.
- *Antidepressant loss of effectiveness:* Sometimes medications become ineffective.
- *Antidepressant-induced suicide:* Especially among 18 to 24-year-olds in early stages of treatment

Selective Serotonin Reuptake Inhibitors (SSRIs)

- Inhibit serotonin reuptake

Tricyclic Antidepressants

- Block reuptake of norepinephrine (and serotonin) at presynaptic neuron
- May take 2 to 4 weeks after first dose to produce desired effect

Monoamine Oxidase Inhibitors (MAOIs)

- MAOIs inhibit the enzyme monoamine oxidase, which is present in the brain, blood platelets, liver, spleen, and kidneys.
- MAOIs are used to treat clients with depression who have not responded to other antidepressant therapies, including electroconvulsive therapy.
- Concurrent use may cause hypertensive crisis with tyramine-containing foods (aged cheese, red wine, pickles, sauerkraut, and smoked meats), amphetamines, antidepressants, dopamine, epinephrine, guanethidine, levodopa, methyldopa, nasal decongestants, norepinephrine, reserpine, or vasoconstrictors.
- Concurrent use with opioid analgesics may cause hypertension or hypotension, coma, or seizures.

Schizophrenia Spectrum and Other Psychotic Disorders

- Group of mental disorders characterized by psychotic features
  - Delusions of persecution: Client believes that he or she is being persecuted by some powerful force.
  - Delusions of grandeur: Client has an exaggerated sense of self that has no basis in reality.
  - Somatic delusions: Client believes that his or her body is changing, which has no basis in reality.
  - Perceptual distortions

- Illusions: Brief experiences of misinterpretation or misperception of reality
- Hallucinations: May be auditory, visual, tactile, olfactory, or gustatory with no basis in reality
  - Safety is the priority.
    — Make sure that client does not have an auditory command telling him or her to harm self or others.

Nursing and Collaborative Management

- Assess for risk of violence to self or others and take appropriate precautions.
- Provide quiet, soothing environment.
- Establish routine and boundaries.
- Provide stable, nonthreatening, and brief social interactions.
- If acting frightened or scared, increase physical space surrounding client and approach calmly.
- Encourage reality-based interests.

Antipsychotic Medications
Traditional Medications

- Treat psychotic behavior

Side Effects
- Extrapyramidal
- Anticholinergic

Nursing Implications
- Encourage fluid (water).
- Gum
- Hard candy
- Increase fiber intake.

Long-Acting Medications
- Promote medication compliance

Side Effects
- Blood dyscrasias
- Neuroleptic malignant syndrome

Nursing Implications
- Change client's position slowly for dizziness.
- Report urinary retention to healthcare provider.

Atypical Medications
- Treat all positive and negative symptoms.

Side Effects
- Multiple side effects, depending on medication

Nursing Implications
- Tolerance to effects usually develops.

Substance Abuse Disorders

Alcohol Abuse
- Alcohol is a central nervous system (CNS) depressant.
  — *Physical dependence:* biological need for alcohol to avoid physical withdrawal symptoms

— *Psychological dependence:* craving for the subjective effect of alcohol
— *Intoxication:* blood alcohol level of 0.1% (100 mg of alcohol per deciliter of blood) or greater

Disulfiram (Antabuse) Therapy

- Alcohol deterrent
- Instruct client to avoid using substances that contain alcohol (e.g., cough medicines, mouthwashes, and aftershave lotions).

Other Medications That Assist With Cravings

- Acamprosate calcium (Campral)
- Naltrexone (ReVia)

Alcohol Withdrawal

- Signs peak after 24 to 48 hours.
- Chlordiazepoxide (Librium) is the most commonly prescribed medication for acute alcohol withdrawal.
- Withdrawal delirium peaks at 48 to 72 hours after cessation of intake and lasts 2 to 3 days.
  - Medical emergency
  - Death can occur from myocardial infarction, fat emboli, peripheral vascular collapse, electrolyte imbalance, aspiration pneumonia, or suicide.

Today's lab report of the lithium level is 1.3 mEq/ml for a client diagnosed with bipolar disorder. Which is the first action the PN should take?
A. Withhold the dose until after breakfast.
B. Give the client the prescribed dose.
C. Obtain a prescription to increase the dose.
D. Withhold the dose and notify charge nurse.

HESI Test Question Approach			
Positive?		YES	NO
Key Words			
Rephrase			
Rule Out Choices			
A	B	C	D

A male client with a history of alcohol abuse is admitted to the medical unit for GI bleeding and pancreatitis. His admission data are BP, 156/96 mm Hg; pulse, 92 beats/min; and temperature, 99.2°F. Which intervention is most important for the nurse to provide?
A. Provide a quiet, low-stimulus environment.
B. Initiate seizure precautions.
C. Administer PRN lorazepam (Ativan) as prescribed.
D. Determine the time and amount of the client's last alcohol intake.

HESI Test Question Approach			
Positive?		YES	NO
Key Words			
Rephrase			
Rule Out Choices			
A	B	C	D

Neurocognitive Disorders

Autism Spectrum Disorder
- Etiology unknown
- Clinical description
  — Hyperactivity
  — Short attention span
  — Impulsivity
  — Aggressivity
  — Self-injurious behaviors
  — Temper tantrums
  — Repetitive mannerisms
  — Preoccupation with objects
  — Spoken language often absent
  — "Islands of genius"
- *Prognosis:* There is no cure for autism. Language skills and intellectual level are the strongest factors related to the prognosis. Only a small percentage of individuals with the disorder go on to live and work independently as adults.

Attention Deficit Hyperactivity Disorder (ADHD)
- Etiology: no known cause, but strong correlation between genetic factors and ADHD
- Clinical description
  — Fidgets when sitting
  — Gets up when expected to stay seated
  — Excessive running when dangerous or inappropriate
  — Loud, disruptive play during quiet activities
  — Forgets and misses appointments
  — Fails to meet deadlines
  — Loses train of conversation
  — Changes topics inappropriately
  — Does not follow rules of games
- Treatment with CNS stimulants may be required to reduce hyperactive behavior and lengthen attention span.
- *Prognosis:* Disorder continues into adolescence in most children. Many adults who had been diagnosed with ADHD as children report a decrease in hyperactivity but continuing difficulty concentrating or attending to complex projects.

Neurocognitive Disorders
Dementia
- Syndrome of progressive deterioration in intellectual functioning secondary to structural or functional changes usually associated with aging; it is not a mental health disorder.
- Marked by loss of long- and short-term memory
- Impairment in judgment, abstract thinking, problem-solving ability, and behavior

Alzheimer's Disease
- Irreversible form of senile dementia caused by nerve cell deterioration; most common type of dementia
- Priority in client care is providing a safe environment.
- Maintain comfort; toilet as necessary; keep dry.

- Reduce environmental stimulation during late afternoon and evening.
- Maintain daily routine.
- Provide environmental cues; turn on lights before dusk; provide night light.
- Provide soothing music.
- Provide reassurance and companionship, especially during difficult evening period.

Medications

- Donepezil (Aricept)
- Galantamine (Razadyne)
- Memantine (Namenda)
- Rivastigmine (Exelon)
- Tacrine (Cognex)

A 68-year-old client diagnosed with Alzheimer's disease, who does not recognize spouse or children and forgets how to eat and dress, is admitted to the nursing home by the PN. What is the PN's priority intervention for the newly admitted client?

A. Establish a daily schedule and routine.
B. Promote involvement in structured activities.
C. Discuss strategies to coordinate care.
D. Stress the importance of nutrition and nurturing.

HESI Test Question Approach			
Positive?		YES	NO
Key Words			
Rephrase			
Rule Out Choices			
A	B	C	D

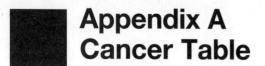

Appendix A
Cancer Table

Type Cancer	Risk Factors/Symptoms	Diagnostics/Classifications	Treatment Options	Nursing Considerations
Leukemia (can be acute or chronic)	The cause, although unknown, is attributed to genetic origin, viral infection, previous treatment with or exposure to radiation, or chemotherapeutic agents.	Blood results and bone marrow examination are the primary methods of diagnosing and classifying the type of leukemia. **Common findings** Decreased platelet count and hemoglobin WBC count to be low, elevated, or excessively elevated Bone marrow biopsy shows immature leukocytes. Chest radiographic examination may show mediastinal lymph node and lung involvement and bone changes. Lymph node biopsy reveals excessive blasts (immature cells). Further studies such as lumbar puncture and CT scan can be performed to determine the presence of leukemic cells outside of the blood and bone marrow. **Classifications of leukemia** Chronic lymphocytic leukemia (CLL): CLL affects lymphoid cells (cells that become lymphocytes, often B cells) and usually grows slowly. It accounts for more than 15,000 new cases of leukemia each year. Most often, people diagnosed with the disease are over age 55. It almost never affects children.	**Acute** Treatment is aimed at eradicating the leukemia with multidrug chemotherapy and/ or bone marrow transplant, and/or hematopoietic stem cell transplantation (HSCT). **Chronic** Treatment is dependent on the kind of cells involved. Medications commonly used include chlorambucil (Leukeran), hydroxyurea, corticosteroids, and cyclophosphamide. Lymph nodes are often irradiated, and blood transfusion may be given if anemia is severe. Although medications are not curative in chronic leukemia, they help to prolong life.	Prevent infections Monitor for bleeding Pain management Encourage a diet high in calories, protein, and vitamins, as well as soft, bland food Monitor for side effects and toxicities of treatment agents Support coping mechanisms

Type Cancer	Risk Factors/Symptoms	Diagnostics/Classifications	Treatment Options	Nursing Considerations
		Chronic myeloid leukemia (CML): CML affects myeloid cells (cells that become any type of blood cell other than lymphocytes) and usually grows slowly at first. It accounts for nearly 5000 new cases of leukemia each year. It mainly affects adults. **Acute lymphocytic (lymphoblastic) leukemia (ALL):** ALL affects lymphoid cells and grows quickly. It accounts for more than 5000 new cases of leukemia each year. ALL is the most common type of leukemia in young children. It also affects adults. **Acute myeloid leukemia (AML):** AML affects myeloid cells and grows quickly. It accounts for more than 13,000 new cases of leukemia each year. It occurs in both adults and children.		
Multiple Myeloma (malignant neoplastic disease of the bone marrow)		Radiographic skeletal studies, bone marrow biopsy, and blood and urine specimens— **monoclonal antibody (M protein)** Common findings include pancytopenia, hypercalcemia, hyperuricemia, and elevated creatinine. **Bence Jones protein** is found in the urine and can result in renal failure.	Treatment is symptom management since multiple myeloma is not curable. Small-dose radiation and chemotherapy may be used; proteasome inhibitors (newer treatment option).	Pain management Prevent infection. Prevent bone injury. Encourage weight-bearing exercises. Encourage 3–4 liters/day. Monitor for side effects of chemotherapy.

(Continued)

Type Cancer	Risk Factors/Symptoms	Diagnostics/Classifications	Treatment Options	Nursing Considerations
Hodgkin's Lymphoma	Occurs twice as often in men as women. Peak targets two primary age ranges: Early adulthood (15–30 years) and around 50 years. No major risk factors but seen commonly in people with mononucleosis, have acquired or congenital immunodeficiency syndromes, those taking immunosuppressive drugs after organ transplantation, those who have been exposed to occupational toxins, or have a genetic predisposition. The presence of HIV increases the incidence of Hodgkin's lymphoma. Symptoms include painless enlargement of the cervical, axillary or inguinal lymph nodes, anorexia, weight loss, fever, night sweats, malaise, and extreme pruritus.	Lymph node biopsy— **Reed Sternberg cell** CXR MRI or PET scan Anemia Low iron, albumin Elevated calcium, alkaline phosphatase **Clinical Staging System for Hodgkin's Disease** **Stage I** • Abnormal single lymph nodes • Regional or single extranodal site **Stage II** • Two or more abnormal lymph nodes on the same side of the diaphragm • Localized involvement of extranodal site and one or more lymph node regions on the same side of the diaphragm **Stage III** • Abnormal lymph node regions on both sides of the diaphragm • May be accompanied by spleen involvement • Now subdivided into lymphatic involvement of the upper abdomen in the spleen (splenic, celiac, and portal nodes) (stage III1) and the lower abdominal nodes in the periaortic, mesenteric, and iliac regions (stage III2) **Stage IV** Diffuse and disseminated involvement of one or more extralymphatic tissues and/or organs—with or without lymph node involvement; the extranodal site is identified as H, hepatic; L, lung; P, pleural; M, marrow; D, dermal; and O, osseous	The stage guides the treatment. Combination chemotherapy for early stage; chemotherapy and radiation for later stages. Bone marrow or peripheral stem cell transplantation (SCT) also considered for later stages.	Skin care Temperature management Monitor for side effects of treatment, therapies. Emotional support

Type Cancer	Risk Factors/Symptoms	Diagnostics/Classifications	Treatment Options	Nursing Considerations
Nonhodgkin's Lymphoma (NHL): (group of malignant neoplasms of primarily B- or T-cell origin, affecting people of all ages) Common names for different types of lymphoma include Burkitt's lymphoma, diffuse large B-cell lymphoma, lymphoblastic lymphoma, and follicular lymphoma.	No known cause but previous infection with human T-cell leukemia/lymphoma virus and the Epstein-Barr virus have been found to be linked to the disease. More common in men over 60 years of age. Symptoms include painless, enlarged lymph nodes and fever, weight loss, night sweats, anemia, pruritus, fatigue. Because of the progression of the disease at the time of diagnosis other symptoms are very possible based on spread (i.e., enlarged liver, pleural effusions, or bone fractures).	Biopsies of lymph nodes, liver, and bone marrow; bone scan, PET scan, MRI CBC Most common staging for NHL—low grade (indolent), intermediate grade (aggressive), and high grade (very aggressive).	Chemotherapy and radiation Monoclonal antibody-rituximab (Rituxan); Ibritumomab (Zevalin) Tumor necrosis factor Interferon therapy	Prevent infections. Monitor for side effects related to treatment therapies.
Brain tumors (can be benign or malignant)	Genetic predisposition Environmental Headache (worse in the morning), dizziness, new onset seizures, change in LOC, personality, or cognition	CT scan (most often used) MRI, PET scan, EEG Stereotactic biopsy,	Surgery (craniotomy/ craniectomy using a surgical navigation system) Chemotherapy/ radiation	Ongoing assessment for changes from baseline or new symptoms Monitor for signs of increased ICP. CSF leakage (meningitis) Infection
Breast	The cause is unknown. Primary risk factors gender (female), age (greater than 50) years, race (North American or Northern European descent), family history (two or more first-degree relatives with the disease, and a first-degree relative with bilateral premenopausal breast cancer), genetics (BRCA1 and BRCA2)	Self-breast exam (>90% of tumors are discovered by the client) Clinical breast exam (a 1 cm tumor is discoverable to physical exam) Mammogram (can detect a 0.5 cm tumor) Biopsy (sentinel lymph node mapping may be used prior to standard lymph node biopsy) MRI, PET scan Estrogen and progesterone receptor status	Treatment based on the type and stage of cancer Radiation, chemotherapy, and surgery alone or in combination may be used. Hormone therapy Tamoxifen Toremifene (Fareston) Letrozole (Femara) Bisphosphonates-pamidronate sodium (Aredia) Raloxifene (Evista) megestrol (Megace)	Clients scheduled for mastectomy: Emotional support (anticipatory grieving; body image acceptance) Wound management Monitor for infection. Hemodynamic stability Post-mastectomy arm exercises Educate about avoiding any procedures involving the arm on the affected side—blood pressure readings, injections, IV infusion of fluids, or the drawing of blood; which may cause edema or infection.

(Continued)

Type Cancer	Risk Factors/Symptoms	Diagnostics/Classifications	Treatment Options	Nursing Considerations
	Breast tumors are usually small, solitary, irregularly shaped, firm, nontender, and nonmobile. There may be a change in skin color, feelings of tenderness, puckering or dimpling of tissue (peau d'orange—skin with the appearance and texture of an orange peel), nipple discharge, retraction of the nipple, and axillary tenderness.		Monoclonal antibody trastuzumab (Herceptin): (used in metastatic breast cancer for clients that express the cancer cell antigen HER2) Bone marrow and stem cell transplantation	Monitoring for side effects of treatment therapies
Cervical	Risk factors linked to sexual behavior (multiple partners and sexually active in teenage years), STIs with several strains of HPV, and to smoking. Vague to no symptoms in the early stages (spotting between menses); vaginal bleeding increasing in amount and with an odor and pain in the back and thighs in the later stages	Pap test; physical examination; colposcopy and cervical biopsy; and additional diagnostic studies, such as a computed tomography (CT) scan, chest radiographic evaluation, IV pyelogram, cystoscopy, sigmoidoscopy, or liver function studies to determine the extent of invasion	Preventative strategies-vaccinations Gardasil; Cervarix Carcinoma in situ—electrocautery, laser, conization, and hysterectomy. Early carcinoma—hysterectomy or intracavitary radiation Late carcinoma—radical hysterectomy with pelvic lymph node dissection; radiation (either external or brachytherapy), chemotherapy (cisplatin-based)	Education about early detection and treatment Pain management Nutritional status Vaginal drainage (amount, color, odor)
Colorectal	Cause unknown Risk factors include age (>50), other disease processes (polyps, ulcerative colitis, and diverticulosis), family history, diet, smoking, excessive intake of alcohol, obesity, and diabetes	Fecal occult blood testing Colonoscopy CT scan Decreased hemoglobin	Radiation Chemotherapy Surgery (bowel resection)	Based on treatment options For client scheduled for surgery with colostomy: Pre-op teaching includes management of bag-barrier device; post-op expectations-change in body image, fears/concerns Stoma should always be pink and moist; mild edema may be expected 1–2 weeks post-op.

Type Cancer	Risk Factors/Symptoms	Diagnostics/Classifications	Treatment Options	Nursing Considerations
Prostate	Onset insidious with the nodule on the posterior portion of the prostate; later symptoms of urinary obstruction and hematuria	Digital rectal examination PSA Biopsy The Gleason grading system Score of 2–4 indicates a slow-progressing tumor. Score of 5–7 indicates a more aggressive tumor.	Radiation (external or brachytherapy) Hormone therapy Luteinizing hormone–releasing hormone (LHRH) agonist—leuprolide (Lupron) and goserelin (Zoladex); LHRH antagonist-Degarelix (Firmagon) Radical prostatectomy	Based on treatment options

From Cooper, K., & Gosnell, K. (2015). *Adult health nursing* (7th ed.). St. Louis, Missouri: Elsevier/Mosby.

Appendix B
Normal Laboratory Values

Test	Adult	Child	Infant/Newborn	Elder	Nursing Implications
Hematological					
Hgb (hemoglobin): mmol/L gm/dL **Possible Critical values <5.0 or >20 g/dL**	Male: 14–18 g/dL or 8.7–11.2 mmol/L (SI units) Female:12–16 g/dL or 7.4–9.9 mmol/L (SI units) Pregnant: 11 g/dL	1–6 yr: 9.5–14 g/dL 6–18 yr: 10–15.5 g/dL	Newborn: 14–24 g/dL 0–2 mo: 12–20 g/dL 2–6 mo: 10–17 g/dL 6 mo-1 yr: 9.5–14 g/dL	Values slightly decreased	High-altitude living increases values. Drug therapy can alter values. Slight Hgb decreases normally occur during pregnancy.
Hct (hematocrit): volume fraction (SI units) or % **Possible Critical values <15% or >60%**	Male: 0.42–0.52 volume fraction (SI units) or (42%–52%) Female: 0.37–0.47 volume fraction or (37%–47%) Pregnant: >33%	1–6 yr: 30–40 6–18 yr: 32–44	Newborn: 44–64 2–8 weeks: 39–59 2–6 months: 35–50 6 mo–1 yr: 29–43	Values slightly decreased	Prolonged stasis from vasoconstriction secondary to the tourniquet can alter values. Abnormalities in RBC size may alter Hct values.
RBC (red blood cell) count: 10^{12}/L (SI units)	Male: 4.7–6.1; Female: 4.2–5.4	1–6 yr: 4–0–5.5 6–18 yr: 4.0–4.5–5	Newborn: 4.8–7.1 2–8 wk: 4–6 2–6 mo: 3.5–5.5 6 mo-yr: 3.5–5.2	Same as adult	Never draw a specimen from an arm with an infusing IV. Exercise and high altitudes can cause an increase in values. Values are usually lower during pregnancy. Drug therapy can alter values.
WBC (white blood cell) count: $\times 10^9$/L (mm^3)	Both genders: 5–10$\times 10^9$/L (SI units) or 5000–10,000 mm^3	≤2 yr: 6.2–17 6200–17,000 mm^3 ≥2 yr: 5–10 5000–10,000 mm^3	Newborn: 9000–30,000 mm^3; Child < 2 years: 6200–17,000 mm^3	Same as adult	Anesthetics, stress, exercise, and convulsions can cause increased values. Drug therapy can decrease values. 24–48 hr postpartum: a count as high as 25,000 is normal.
Platelet count: $\times 10^9$/L (mm^3)	Both genders: 150–400 (150,000–400,000 mm^3)	150–400 (150,000–400,000 mm^3)	Premature infant: 100–300 (100,000–300,000 mm^3);	Same as adult	Living at high altitudes, exercising strenuously, or taking oral contraceptives may increase values.

Test	Adult	Child	Infant/Newborn	Elder	Nursing Implications
			Newborn: 150–300 (150,000–300,000 mm^3); Infant: 200–475 (200,000–475,000 mm^3)		Decreased values may be caused by hemorrhage, DIC, reduced production of platelets, infections, use of prosthetic heart valves, and drugs (e.g., acetaminophen, aspirin, chemotherapy, H$_2$ blockers, INH, Levaquin, streptomycin, sulfonamides, and thiazide diuretics).

HESI Hint: The laboratory values that are most important to know for the NCLEX-RN exam are Hgb, Hct, WBCs, Na$^+$, K$^+$, BUN, blood glucose, ABGs (arterial blood gases), bilirubin for newborns, and therapeutic range for PT and PTT.

Test	Adult	Child	Infant/Newborn	Elder	Nursing Implications
SED rate, ESR (erythrocyte sedimentation rate): mm/hr	Male: up to 15; Female: up to 20; Pregnant (all trimesters): up to 10	Same as adult	Newborn: 0–2	Same as adult	Pregnancy (second and third trimester) can cause elevations in ESR.
PT (prothrombin time): sec	Both genders: 11–12.5; Pregnant: slight ↓	Same as adult	Same as adult	Same as adult	PT is used to help regulate warfarin (Coumadin) dosages. Therapeutic range: 1.5–2 times normal or control.
PTT (partial thromboplastin time): sec (see APTT, below)	Both genders: 60–70; Pregnant: slight ↓	Same as adult	Same as adult	Same as adult	PTT is used to help regulate heparin dosages. Therapeutic range: 1.5–2.5 times normal or control.
INR (international normalized ratio)	Both genders: 0.8–1.2	Same as adult	Same as adult	Same as adult	Ideal INR value must be individualized. Typical values for certain clients: Values for clients with atrial fibrillation and deep vein thrombosis are between 2.0 and 3.0; values for clients with mechanical heart valves are between 3.0 and 4.0.
APTT (activated partial thromboplastin time): sec	Both genders: 30–40	Same as adult	Same as adult	Same as adult	APTT is used to help partially regulate heparin dosages. Therapeutic range: 1.5–2.5 times normal or control.

(Continued)

Test	Adult	Child	Infant/Newborn	Elder	Nursing Implications
Blood Chemistry					

Alkaline phosphatase: U/L	Both genders: 35–120	1–3 yr: 185–383
		4–6 yr: 191–450
		7–9 yr: 218–499
		10–11 yr:
		Male: 174–624;
		   Female: 169–657
		12–13 yr:
		Male: 245–584;
		Female: 141–499
		14–15 yr:
		Male: 169–618;
		   Female: 103–283
		16–19 yr:
		Male: 98–317;
		Female: 82–169
				Slightly higher than adult	Hemolysis of specimen can cause falsely elevated values.

Albumin: g/dL	Both genders: 35–50 (3.5–5) Pregnant: slight ↓	40–59 (4.5–9)	Premature infant: 30–42 (3–4.2); Newborn: 35–54 (3.5–5.4); Infant: 44–54 (4.4–5.4)	Same as adult	No special preparation is needed.
Bilirubin total: mg/dL	Total: 0.3–1 Indirect: 0.2–0.8 Direct: 0.1–0.3	Same as adult	Newborn: 1–12	Same as adult	Client is kept NPO, except for water, for 8–12 hr before testing. Prevent hemolysis of blood during venipuncture. Do not shake tube; this can cause inaccurate values. Protect blood sample from bright light.
Hematological					
Calcium: mmol/L (mg/dL)	Both genders: 2.25–2.75 (9–10.5)	2.2–2.7 (8.8–10.8)	<10 days: 1.9–2.60 (7.6–10.4); Cord: 2.25–2.88 (9–11.5); 10 days-2 yr: 2.3–2.65 (9–10.6)	Values tend to decrease.	No special preparation is needed. Use of thiazide diuretics can cause increased calcium values.
Chloride: mmol/L (mEq/L)	Both genders: 98–106	90–110	Newborn: 96–106; Premature infant: 95–110	Same as adult	Do not collect from an arm with an infusing IV solution.
Cholesterol: mmol/L (mg/dL)	Both genders: <5.0 (<200)	10–11 yr: Male: 3.10–5.90 (120–228); Female: 3.16–6.26 (122–242)	Infant (7–12 mo): Male: 2.15–5.30 (83–205); Female: 1.76–5.59 (68–216) Newborn (0–1 mo): Male: 0.98–4.50 (38–174); Female: 1.45–5.04 (56–195)	Same as adult	Do not collect from an arm with an infusing IV solution.

Test	Adult	Child	Infant/Newborn	Elder	Nursing Implications
CPK (creatine phosphokinase): IU/L	Male: 55–170; Female: 30–135	Same as adult	Newborn: 65–580	Same as adult	Specimen must not be stored before running test.
Creatinine: mcmol/L (mg/dL)	Male: 53–106 (0.6–1.2); Female: 44–97 (0.5–1.1)	Child/Adolescent (1–18 yr): 18–62 (0.2–0.7)	Newborn (0–1 week): 53–97 (0.6–1.1); Infant (7 days-12 mo): 18–35 (0.2–0.4)	Decrease in muscle mass may cause decreased values.	NPO for 8 hr before testing is preferred but not required. BUN-to-creatinine ratio of 20:1 indicates adequate kidney functioning.
Glucose: mmol/L (mg/dL)	Both genders: 4–6 (36–108)	≤2 yr: 3.3–5.5 (60–100) >2 yr: <6.1 (70–110)	Cord: 2.5–5.3 (45–96); Premature infant: 1.1–3.3 (20–60) Neonate: (0–28 days): 1.7–3.3 (30–60); Infant (1 mo-2 yr): 2.2–5.0 (40–90) Newborn/Infant: 16–24	Normal range increases after age 50.	Client is kept NPO, except for water, for 8 hr before testing. Stress, infection, and caffeine can cause increased values.
HCO$_3$−: mmol/L (mEq/L)	Both genders: 21–28	21–28	Newborn 13–22; Infant: 20–28	Same as adult	None
Iron: mcmol/L (mcg/dL)	Male: 14–32 (80–180); Female: 11–29 (60–160)	Child 4–10 yr: Male: 2.7–22.9 (15–128); Female: 5.0–21.8 (28–122)	Newborn: Male: 12.9–36.3 (72–203); Female: 13.4–42.1 (75–235)	Same as adult	NPO for 8 hr before test is preferred but not required.
TIBC (total iron binding capacity): mcmol/L (mcg/dL)	Both genders: 45–82 (250–460)	Same as adult	Newborn: 16.8–41.5 (94–232)	Same as adult	None
LDH (lactic dehydrogenase): U/L	Both genders: 100–190	60–170	Newborn: 160–450; Infant: 100–250	Same as adult	Do not give IM injections for 8–12 hr before test. Hemolysis of blood causes a false-positive result.
Potassium: mmol/L (mEq/L)	Both genders: 3.5–5	3.4–4.7	Newborn: 3.9–5.9; Infant: 4.1–5.3	Same as adult	Hemolysis of specimen can result in falsely elevated values. Exercise of the forearm with tourniquet in place may cause an increased potassium level.
Protein total: g/L (g/dL)	Both genders: 64–83 (6.4–8.3)	62–80 (6.2–8)	Premature infant: 42–76 (4.2–7.6); Newborn: 46–74 (4.6–7.4); Infant: 60–67 (6–6.7)	Same as adult	NPO for 8 hr before test is preferred but not required.
AST/SGOT (aspartate aminotransferase): U/L	0–35 Female slightly lower than adult male	3–6 yr: 15–50 6–12 yr: 10–50 12–18 yr: 10–40	0–5 days: 35–140 <3 yr: 15–60	Slightly higher than adult	Hemolysis of specimen can result in falsely elevated values. Exercise may cause an increased value.

(Continued)

Test	Adult	Child	Infant/Newborn	Elder	Nursing Implications
ALT/SGPT (alanine aminotransferase): U/mL	Both genders: 4–36	Similar to adult	Values may be 2× as high as an adult's value.	Slightly higher than adult	Hemolysis of specimen can result in falsely elevated values. Exercise may cause an increased value.
Sodium: mEq/L	Both genders: 136–145	136–145	Newborn: 134–144; Infant: 134–150	Same as adult	Do not collect from an arm with an infusing IV solution.
Triglycerides: mmol/L (mg/dL)	Male: 0.45–1.81 (40–160); Female: 0.40–1.52 (35–135)	4–6 yr: Male: 0.36–1.31 (32–116); Female: 0.36–1.31 (32–116) 7–9 yr: Male: 0.32–1.46 (28–129); Female: 0.32–1.46 (28–129) 10–11 yr: Male: 0.27–1.55 (24–137); Female: 0.44–1.58 (39–140) 12–13 yr: Male: 0.27–1.64 (24–145); Female: 0.42–1.47 (37–130) 14–15 yr: Male: 0.38–1.86 (34–165); Female: 0.43–1.52 (38–135) 16–19 yr: Male: 0.38–1.58 (34–140); Female: 0.42–1.58 (37–140)	0–3 yr: Male: 0.31–1.41 (27–125); Female: 0.31–1.41 (27–125)	Same as adult	Client is kept NPO for 12 hr before test. No alcohol for 24 hr before test.
BUN (blood urea nitrogen): mmol/L (mg/dL)	Both genders: 36–7.1 (10–20)	1.8–6.4 (5–18)	Newborn: 0.7–4.6 (2–13); Cord: 7.5–14.3 (21–40); Infant: 1.8–6.0 (5–17)	Slightly higher	None
Arterial Blood Chemistry					
pH	Both genders: 7.35–7.45	Child >2 yr: Same as adult	Newborn: 7.32–7.49; 2 mo-2 yr: 7.34–7.46	Same as adult	Specimen must be heparinized. Specimen must be iced for transport. All air bubbles must be expelled from sample. Direct pressure to puncture site must be maintained.

Test	Adult	Child	Infant/Newborn	Elder	Nursing Implications
PCO_2: mm Hg	Both genders: 35–45	Same as adult	<2 yr: 26–41	Same as adult	Specimen must be heparinized. Specimen must be iced for transport. All air bubbles must be expelled from sample. Direct pressure to puncture site must be maintained.
PO_2: mm Hg	Both genders: 80–100	Same as adult	Newborn/Infant: 16–24	Same as adult	Specimen must be heparinized. Specimen must be iced for transport. All air bubbles must be expelled from sample. Direct pressure to puncture site must be maintained.
HCO_3-: mmol/L (mEq/L)	Both genders: 21–28	Same as adult	Newborn/Infant: 16–24	Same as adult	Specimen must be heparinized. Specimen must be iced for transport. All air bubbles must be expelled from sample. Direct pressure to puncture site must be maintained.
O_2 saturation: %	Both genders: 95–100	Same as adult	Newborn: 40–90	95	Specimen must be heparinized. Specimen must be iced for transport. All air bubbles must be expelled from sample. Direct pressure to puncture site must be maintained.

BUN, blood urea nitrogen; *DIC,* disseminated intravascular coagulation; *DVT,* deep vein thrombosis; *IM,* intramuscular; *INH,* isoniazid; *NPO,* nothing by mouth; *PCO$_2$,* carbon dioxide partial pressure; *PO$_2$,* oxygen partial pressure; *HCO$_3$–,* bicarbonate.
From Pagana, T. J., & Pagana, K. D. (2013). *Mosby's Canadian manual of diagnostic and laboratory tests* (1st ed.). Toronto: Mosby; Pagana, T. J., & Pagana, K. D. (2013). *Mosby's manual of diagnostic and laboratory tests* (11th ed.). St Louis: Mosby.

Appendix C
Comparison of Three Types of Hepatitis

Characteristics	Hepatitis A (Infectious Hepatitis)	Hepatitis B (Serum Hepatitis)	Hepatitis C
Source of Infection	• Contaminated food • Contaminated water or shellfish	• Contaminated blood products • Contaminated needles or surgical instruments • Mother to child at birth	• Contaminated blood products • Contaminated needles • IV drug use • Dialysis
Route of Infection	• Oral • Fecal • Parenteral • Person to person	• Parenteral • Oral • Fecal • Direct contact • Breast milk • Sexual contact	• Parenteral • Sexual contact
Incubation Period	15–50 days	14–180 days	14–180 days (average)
Onset	Abrupt	Insidious	Insidious
Seasonal Variation	• Autumn • Winter	All year	All year
Age Group Affected	• Children • Young adults	Any age	Any age
Vaccine	Yes	Yes	No
Inoculation	Yes	Yes	Yes
Potential for Chronic Liver Disease	No	Yes	Yes
Immunity	Yes	Yes	No
Treatment	• Prevention—hepatitis A (HAV) vaccine • Proper handwashing • Avoid contaminated food or water. • Obtain immunoglobulin within 14 days if exposed to the virus.	• Prevention—hepatitis B (HBV) vaccine for high-risk groups • Antiviral and immunomodulating drugs	• Subcutaneous pegylated interferon alpha once a week and oral ribavirin (Copegus, Rebetol) daily
Complications	Very few	• Chronic hepatitis • Cirrhosis • Hepatitis D • Liver cancer	• Chronic hepatitis • Cirrhosis • Liver cancer

Appendix D
Compare and Contrast: Parkinson's Disease, Myasthenia Gravis, and Multiple Sclerosis

	Parkinson's Disease	Myasthenia Gravis	Multiple Sclerosis
Definition	Chronic, progressive neurodegenerative disorder	Autoimmune disorder of neuromuscular junction with fluctuating weakness of some skeletal muscles	Chronic, progressive, degenerative disorder Demyelination of nerve fibers of the brain and spinal cord
Patient	Peak onset in 70s, men	Onset between 10 and 65, women more common	Young to middle age, female, temperate climates
Etiology	Unknown but with genetic and environmental components	Antibodies attack acetylcholine receptors, which prevents stimulation of muscle contraction	Unknown; may be related to viral, immunologic, and genetic factors.
Signs and Symptoms	Gradual, insidious; may be unilateral; tremor more pronounced at rest Rigidity, bradykinesia, stooped posture, drooling, masked face, shuffling gait, and jerky movements	Fluctuating weakness of skeletal muscles; strength restored after period of rest Primarily muscles of the eyes, mouth, and respiratory system Highly variable disorder	Insidious, gradual onset Remissions and exacerbations: limb weakness, diplopia, numbness, tingling, and neuropathic pain Decreased bowel, bladder function Sexual dysfunction Short term memory and cognitive changes
Nursing Management	Maximize neurologic function Maintain independence in ADL Optimize psychosocial aspects Safety	Optimize endurance Manage fatigue Avoid complications Maintain quality of life Safety	Maintain independence in ADL Maximize neuromuscular function Manage disabling fatigue Optimize psychosocial adjustment to illness Reduce exacerbating factors Safety
Medications	Dopaminergics Anticholinergics Antihistamine Monoamine oxidase inhibitors (MAIOs) Catechol-*O*-methyltransferase (COMT) inhibitors	Anticholinesterase drugs Corticosteroids Immunosuppressants	Corticosteroids Immunomodulators Cholinergics, anticholinergics Muscle relaxants Acetylcholinesterase inhibitors

ADL, activities of daily living

NCLEX-PN® Examination Practice Questions

Management

1. Which activity should the practical nurse (PN) delegate to unlicensed assistive personnel (UAP)? (Select all that apply.)
   A. Observe a client to see whether he can hear better after discontinuation (DC) of an IV antibiotic.
   B. Encourage additional oral fluids to an elderly client with pneumonia.
   C. Report the ability of a client to eat the meal on the supper tray unassisted.
   D. Record the number of liquid stools of a client who has received lactulose.
   F. Take the vital signs of clients scheduled for early morning tests.

HESI Test Question Approach		
Positive?	YES	NO
Key Words		
Rephrase		
Rule Out Choices		
A	B	C	D	E

2. The PN is caring for a group of patients with the assistance of several UAPs. Which situation requires an intervention by the PN?
   A. The client with active tuberculosis who is leaving his room without a mask
   B. The client with pneumonia and dehydration who has not had anything to drink for 4 hours
   C. The client with asthma who complains of being anxious and unable to concentrate
   D. The client who is a high fall risk and is trying to go to the bathroom

HESI Test Question Approach		
Positive?	YES	NO
Key Words		
Rephrase		
Rule Out Choices		
A	B	C	D

3. The PN reports that a hospitalized client has threatened to cut herself. In what order should the PN implement the following actions? (Place them in order, first to last.)
   A. Perform a sweep of the room and remove any cords or sharp objects.
   B. Call the charge nurse and ask for an additional UAP.
   C. Stay with the client until a UAP is assigned to sit with client.
   D. Continue to establish rapport and ensure confidentiality.

HESI Test Question Approach		
Positive?	YES	NO
Key Words		
Rephrase		
Rule Out Choices		
A	B	C	D

4. The UAP is assisting with the care of several clients on a postpartum unit. Which assignment should the PN delegate to the UAP?
   A. Assess fundal firmness and lochia for the clients who delivered vaginally.
   B. Take vital signs every 15 minutes for a client with preeclampsia.
   C. Provide breastfeeding instructions for a primigravida.
   D. Assist with daily care activities for the clients on bed rest.

HESI Test Question Approach			
Positive?		YES	NO
Key Words			
Rephrase			
Rule Out Choices			
A	B	C	D

Advanced Clinical Concepts

5. Which client is at the highest risk for developing respiratory complications?
   A. A 21-year-old with dehydration and cerebral palsy who is dependent in daily activities
   B. A 60-year-old who has had type 2 diabetes for 20 years and was admitted with cellulitis
   C. An obese 30-year-old with hypertension who is noncompliant with the medication regimen
   D. A 40-year-old with a serum K^+ of 3.4 mEq/L, who is taking a loop diuretic and complains of fatigue

HESI Test Question Approach			
Positive?		YES	NO
Key Words			
Rephrase			
Rule Out Choices			
A	B	C	D

6. A PN is administering medications to a client with a history of substance abuse admitted for an overdose. Which interventions are priorities to include in this client's plan of care? (Select all that apply.)
   A. Allow the client to take his or her medications independently.
   B. Ensure that all medications have been swallowed before leaving the client's room.
   C. Request that oral pain medications be changed from tablet to oral suspension.
   D. Give flumazenil every 6 hours around the clock.
   E. Only give medications to the client via the intravenous route.

HESI Test Question Approach				
Positive?			YES	NO
Key Words				
Rephrase				
Rule Out Choices				
A	B	C	D	E

7. A postoperative client has received normal saline intravenously at 125 mL/hr. The PN observes a dark yellow urine output. The first hour the output was 50 mL; the next hour, it was 32 mL; and the third hour, it was 28 mL. What action should the PN take?
   A. Give a bolus with ½ NS at 200 mL/hr.
   B. Inform the registered nurse.
   C. Monitor output for another 2 hours.
   D. Draw samples for the BUN and creatinine labs.

HESI Test Question Approach		
Positive?	**YES**	**NO**
Key Words		
Rephrase		
Rule Out Choices		
A	B	C	D

8. A 54-year-old male client was admitted to the acute care unit after a stapling of his esophageal varices. What intervention should the PN expect to be a part of this client's plan of care?
   A. Frequent oral suctioning
   B. Bleeding precautions
   C. Diet high in protein
   D. Complete bed rest

HESI Test Question Approach		
Positive?	**YES**	**NO**
Key Words		
Rephrase		
Rule Out Choices		
A	B	C	D

9. A client's arterial blood gas results are pH, 7.29; P_{CO_2}, 55 mm Hg; and HCO_3, 26 mEq/L. Which is the correct interpretation of these values?
   A. Normal blood gas values
   B. Respiratory acidosis
   C. Respiratory alkalosis
   D. Metabolic acidosis

HESI Test Question Approach		
Positive?	**YES**	**NO**
Key Words		
Rephrase		
Rule Out Choices		
A	B	C	D

10. A client who has chronic back pain is not receiving adequate pain relief from an oral analgesic. Which alternative action should the PN explore to promote the client's independence?
   A. Encourage the client to take the maximum dosage.
   B. Obtain a prescription for an adjuvant medication.
   C. Consider the client's receptivity to complementary therapy.
   D. Encourage counseling to prevent future addiction.

HESI Test Question Approach			
Positive?		**YES**	**NO**
Key Words			
Rephrase			
Rule Out Choices			
A	**B**	**C**	**D**

Maternal-Newborn Nursing

11. A client at 41 weeks' gestation who is in active labor calls the PN to report that her membranes have ruptured. The PN views the perineum and sees the cord. Which action should the PN implement first?
   A. Place the client in a knee-chest position.
   B. Cover the cord with sterile, warm, saline gauze.
   C. Assist with preparing for an emergency cesarean birth.
   D. Start oxygen by face mask at 10 L/min.

HESI Test Question Approach			
Positive?		**YES**	**NO**
Key Words			
Rephrase			
Rule Out Choices			
A	**B**	**C**	**D**

12. A client at 39 weeks' gestation plans to have an epidural block when labor is established. What intervention should the nurse implement to prevent side effects?
   A. Reinforce teaching about the effects of the epidural.
   B. Place the client in a chair next to the bed with her feet elevated.
   C. Continuously monitor the fetal heart rate and contractions.
   D. Assist the client to empty her bladder every 2 hours.

HESI Test Question Approach			
Positive?		**YES**	**NO**
Key Words			
Rephrase			
Rule Out Choices			
A	**B**	**C**	**D**

13. A client whose last menses was 6 weeks ago presents in the clinic with right lower quadrant abdominal pain, no vaginal bleeding, and pain in her right shoulder. Which action should the PN take first?
   A. Check for abdominal rebound tenderness, distention, and fever.
   B. Obtain a full set of vital signs and assist with IV access.
   C. Observe client for recent musculoskeletal injury, bruising, or abuse.
   D. Collect specimens for pregnancy test, hemoglobin, and WBC.

HESI Test Question Approach			
Positive?		YES	NO
Key Words			
Rephrase			
Rule Out Choices			
A	B	C	D

14. A pregnant client with a low hematocrit and low hemoglobin asks the PN why she should take her iron supplement. Which explanation should the PN offer?
   A. Iron promotes collagen production, which aids healing during the postpartum period.
   B. Iron reduces the risk of preterm labor.
   C. Replacing iron through the diet alone is difficult.
   D. Additional iron is necessary to replace the blood lost during delivery.

HESI Test Question Approach			
Positive?		YES	NO
Key Words			
Rephrase			
Rule Out Choices			
A	B	C	D

Medical-Surgical Review

15. A client is returning to the unit after an intravenous pyelogram (IVP). Which intervention should the PN include in the plan of care?
   A. Maintain bed rest.
   B. Increase fluid intake.
   C. Monitor for hematuria.
   D. Continue NPO status.

HESI Test Question Approach			
Positive?		YES	NO
Key Words			
Rephrase			
Rule Out Choices			
A	B	C	D

16. A female client has chronic urinary tract infections. The PN is reinforcing teaching to the client about a prescription for ciprofloxacin 500 mg PO bid. What side effect(s) could the client expect over the course of medication therapy? (Select all that apply.)
    A. Photosensitivity
    B. Dyspepsia
    C. Diarrhea
    D. Urinary frequency
    E. Anemia

HESI Test Question Approach			
Positive?		YES	NO
Key Words			
Rephrase			
Rule Out Choices			
A	B	C	D	E

17. A PN working on a hospice unit finds a client crying. The client states that he is afraid to die. Which actions should the PN implement? (Select all that apply.)
    A. Sit quietly with the client and listen to his concerns.
    B. Provide the client with privacy.
    C. Administer an antianxiety medication to the client.
    D. Ask client's permission to contact a spiritual counselor or minister.
    E. Assess the client for signs of impending death.

HESI Test Question Approach			
Positive?		YES	NO
Key Words			
Rephrase			
Rule Out Choices			
A	B	C	D	E

18. A client with a peritoneal dialysis catheter calls the clinic to report that he feels poorly and seems to have a fever. What is the PN's best response?
    A. Encourage the client to come to the clinic that day to be evaluated.
    B. Instruct the client to increase his fluid intake to 3 L/day.
    C. Review the client's peritoneal dialysis regimen.
    D. Ask about the client's recent dietary intake of protein and iron.

HESI Test Question Approach			
Positive?		YES	NO
Key Words			
Rephrase			
Rule Out Choices			
A	B	C	D

19. A client is admitted with chest pain. Which assessment finding(s) should be reported to the charge nurse immediately? (Select all that apply.)
   A. Diaphoresis
   B. Irregular heart rate
   C. Elevated troponin level
   D. Radiating jaw pain
   E. O_2 saturation of 93%

HESI Test Question Approach			
Positive?		**YES**	**NO**
Key Words			
Rephrase			
Rule Out Choices			

A	B	C	D	E

20. The PN is reviewing the discharge instructions with a client who has a history of angina. Which instruction should the PN emphasize as the most important?
   A. Avoid activity that requires the Valsalva maneuver.
   B. Seek emergency treatment if chest pain persists after the third nitroglycerin dose.
   C. Rest for 30 minutes after having chest pain before resuming activity.
   D. Keep extra nitroglycerin in an airtight, light-resistant bottle.

HESI Test Question Approach			
Positive?		**YES**	**NO**
Key Words			
Rephrase			
Rule Out Choices			

A	B	C	D

21. The PN is reviewing the medication diltiazem with a client. Which dietary recommendation should be included?
   A. Maintain a low-sodium diet.
   B. Eat a banana each morning.
   C. Eat high-fiber foods daily.
   D. Avoid grapefruit products.

HESI Test Question Approach			
Positive?		**YES**	**NO**
Key Words			
Rephrase			
Rule Out Choices			

A	B	C	D

22. A female client with a history of Raynaud's disease wants to know how to manage her symptoms. What teaching should the PN reinforce?
    A. Take oral analgesic at regularly spaced intervals.
    B. Avoid extremes of heat and cold.
    C. Limit intake of foods and fluids with caffeine.
    D. Keep involved extremities in a dependent position.

HESI Test Question Approach			
Positive?		**YES**	**NO**
Key Words			
Rephrase			
Rule Out Choices			
A	**B**	**C**	**D**

23. The PN is providing care for a client admitted with thrombocytopenia. Which problem should the PN immediately report to the charge nurse?
    A. Bleeding gums
    B. Refusing breakfast
    C. Complaints of insomnia
    D. Constant fatigue

HESI Test Question Approach			
Positive?		**YES**	**NO**
Key Words			
Rephrase			
Rule Out Choices			
A	**B**	**C**	**D**

24. A client who is admitted with cancer of the larynx is scheduled for a laryngectomy tomorrow. What client education should the PN review with him tonight?
    A. Anticipated body image changes
    B. Pain management expectations
    C. Communication techniques
    D. Postoperative nutritional needs

HESI Test Question Approach			
Positive?		**YES**	**NO**
Key Words			
Rephrase			
Rule Out Choices			
A	**B**	**C**	**D**

25. **A victim of a motor vehicle collision is dead on arrival at the emergency department. Which action should the nurse take to assist the spouse?**
    A. Ask whether there are relatives, friends, or clergy to call.
    B. Talk about the former relationship with the spouse.
    C. Provide education about the stages of grief and loss.
    D. Assess the spouse's level of anxiety.

HESI Test Question Approach			
Positive?		YES	NO
Key Words			
Rephrase			
Rule Out Choices			
A	B	C	D

26. **The PN is interviewing a client in the prenatal clinic for violence during pregnancy. Which statement(s) describe(s) an appropriate technique to assess for violence? (Select all that apply.)**
    A. Women should be assessed only if they are members of a high-risk group.
    B. Women may be assessed in the presence of young children.
    C. Women should be assessed once during pregnancy.
    D. As the pregnancy progresses, women should be reassessed face to face by a nurse.
    E. Women should be assessed alone (i.e., without the intimate partner).

HESI Test Question Approach				
Positive?			YES	NO
Key Words				
Rephrase				
Rule Out Choices				
A	B	C	D	E

27. **The PN reminds several clients on the mental health unit that breakfast is at 0800, medications are given at 0900, and group therapy sessions begin at 1000. Which treatment modality has been implemented?**
    A. Milieu therapy
    B. Behavior modification
    C. Peer therapy
    D. Problem-solving

HESI Test Question Approach			
Positive?		YES	NO
Key Words			
Rephrase			
Rule Out Choices			
A	B	C	D

28. The PN is taking a client to the x-ray department. As the nurse starts to enter the elevator with him, the client becomes panic-stricken and states, "I can't do this." Which intervention should the PN implement first?
   A. Ask one more staff member to ride in the elevator.
   B. Offer an antianxiety medication.
   C. Begin desensitization about riding the elevator.
   D. Affirm his fears about riding the elevator.

HESI Test Question Approach			
Positive?		YES	NO
Key Words			
Rephrase			
Rule Out Choices			
A	B	C	D

29. A male client who has been diagnosed with post-traumatic stress disorder is found one night trying to strangle his roommate. Which interventions should the PN implement immediately? (Select all that apply.)
   A. Give the client a sedative.
   B. Ask the victim to share his feelings.
   C. Move the client to a private room.
   D. Place the client in restraints.
   E. Assign a UAP to sit with the client.

HESI Test Question Approach				
Positive?			YES	NO
Key Words				
Rephrase				
Rule Out Choices				
A	B	C	D	E

30. The PN is providing care for a client with a borderline personality disorder who is being manipulative. Which intervention should the PN expect to see in the client's plan of care?
   A. Refer the client's requests to one nurse.
   B. Do not challenge inappropriate behavior.
   C. Limit the client's contact with other clients.
   D. Remove consequences for acting-out behaviors.

HESI Test Question Approach			
Positive?		YES	NO
Key Words			
Rephrase			
Rule Out Choices			
A	B	C	D

31. An adolescent client, admitted to the mental health unit for anorexia nervosa, frequently isolates herself. What is the PN's priority intervention?
A. Teach the client the importance of self-expression.
B. Monitor the client's activities closely.
C. Include the client in daily group therapy.
D. Facilitate social interactions with others.

HESI Test Question Approach

Positive?			YES	NO
Key Words				
Rephrase				
Rule Out Choices				
A	B		C	D

32. The PN is planning the daily schedule for clients on the mental health unit. A client who is manic should be encouraged to participate in which group activity?
A. A basketball game in the gym
B. Jogging at least 1 mile
C. A Ping-Pong game with a peer
D. A group activity with the art therapist

HESI Test Question Approach

Positive?			YES	NO
Key Words				
Rephrase				
Rule Out Choices				
A	B		C	D

Delegation and Prioritization

33. A PN is making client assignments for the night shift. The nursing team has another PN and two UAPs. Which duties could be delegated to the UAPs? (Select all that apply.)
A. Transport a client who has had a stroke to the radiology department for a chest radiograph.
B. Reinforce the technique for insulin injection to a client newly diagnosed with diabetes.
C. Bathe a 25-year-old client who is a quadriplegic and has a large, stage IV pressure ulcer.
D. Turn a 92-year-old client with end-stage heart failure who has a DNR order.
E. Inform family members in clients' rooms that visiting hours are over.

HESI Test Question Approach

Positive?				YES	NO
Key Words					
Rephrase					
Rule Out Choices					
A	B	C	D	E	

34. **A hospitalized client has type 2 diabetes. Which task(s) for this client can the PN delegate to the UAP? (Select all that apply.)**
    A. Notifying the dietitian of a prescribed consult
    B. Reporting the client's insulin injection technique
    C. Obtaining the finger stick blood glucose level before meals
    D. Reminding the client to dry the toes carefully after a shower
    E. Talking with the client about foods that raise the blood glucose level

HESI Test Question Approach			
Positive?		YES	NO
Key Words			
Rephrase			
Rule Out Choices			
A	B	C	D	E

35. **After a change-of-shift report, the PN reviews her assignments. Which client should the PN assess first?**
    A. An elderly client receiving palliative care for heart failure who complains of constipation and nervousness
    B. A client admitted for possible pneumonia with a heart rate of 110 and a respiratory rate of 24
    C. A middle-aged client with end-stage renal failure whose urinary output is 95 mL over 8 hours
    D. A client taking Coumadin who is receiving oxygen at 3 L/min and whose respiratory rate is 12/min

HESI Test Question Approach			
Positive?		YES	NO
Key Words			
Rephrase			
Rule Out Choices			
A	B	C	D

36. **The female PN has been assigned to care for a male Muslim client. Which actions would demonstrate cultural sensitivity? (Select all that apply.)**
    A. Cover her hair with a cloth when going into the patient's room.
    B. Ask a male UAP to assist the client with his bath.
    C. Move the bed to face the east.
    D. Ensure that there is no pork in his food.
    E. Provide the client with a new ostomy bag before each prayer time.

HESI Test Question Approach			
Positive?		YES	NO
Key Words			
Rephrase			
Rule Out Choices			
A	B	C	D	E

37. The PN enters the exam room after a client has been told by her healthcare provider that she has advanced ovarian cancer. How should the PN respond?

A. Share with the client information about survivor rates.

B. Discuss with the client the different treatment protocols.

C. Encourage the client to get a second opinion.

D. Sit quietly with the client and allow her to share her feelings.

HESI Test Question Approach		
Positive?	**YES**	**NO**
Key Words		
Rephrase		
Rule Out Choices		
A	B	C	D

38. Which assessment finding indicates the expected outcome of administering donepezil to a client with Alzheimer's disease?

A. Increased muscle strength and tone

B. Fewer episodes of urinary incontinence

C. Increased ability to solve simple problems

D. Improved appetite, which supports weight gain

HESI Test Question Approach		
Positive?	**YES**	**NO**
Key Words		
Rephrase		
Rule Out Choices		
A	B	C	D

39. In caring for an older client with dementia who has sundowning syndrome, which intervention(s) should the PN implement? (Select all that apply.)

A. Observe for tiredness at the end of the day.

B. Maintain a quiet unit during the late afternoon.

C. Monitor for medication side effects.

D. Assess for decreased gross motor movement.

E. Reorient the client to reality.

HESI Test Question Approach			
Positive?		**YES**	**NO**
Key Words			
Rephrase			
Rule Out Choices			
A	B	C	D	E

40. The PN starts to help an elderly male client with dementia get out of bed. The client becomes angry and yells at the nurse, "Get out of here! I'll get up when I'm ready." Which action by the nurse is most likely to be helpful in reducing the client's agitation?
    A. Continue to encourage the client to get out of bed.
    B. Explain why ambulation is important.
    C. Acknowledge how he feels but continue to get him out of bed.
    D. Return in 30 minutes and try again.

HESI Test Question Approach			
Positive?		YES	NO
Key Words			
Rephrase			
Rule Out Choices			
A	B	C	D

41. A client with diabetes is admitted for osteomyelitis. Which regimen for hypoglycemic control would the PN expect the healthcare provider to prescribe for this client?
    A. Supplemental scale using regular insulin alone
    B. Continue home oral hypoglycemic medications
    C. An alpha-glucosidase inhibitor
    D. A combination of long-acting and short-acting insulin

HESI Test Question Approach			
Positive?		YES	NO
Key Words			
Rephrase			
Rule Out Choices			
A	B	C	D

42. The PN is making a home visit to provide wound care for an 80-year-old man and suspects that the client is being physically abused. Which intervention should the PN implement first?
    A. Notify the RN case manager.
    B. Confront the caregiver.
    C. Call the police.
    D. Ask the client to validate the abuse.

HESI Test Question Approach			
Positive?		YES	NO
Key Words			
Rephrase			
Rule Out Choices			
A	B	C	D

43. The PN is working on a hospice unit. A client is resting quietly but moans when turned. The family has asked the nurse for more pain medication for the client. How should the PN respond?
   A. Discuss with the family why they believe the client needs more pain medication.
   B. Ask the family to leave to allow the client to rest.
   C. Since the client is in hospice care, give the medication as the family requests.
   D. Ask the charge nurse to request a prescription for a sedative for the client.

HESI Test Question Approach			
Positive?		YES	NO
Key Words			
Rephrase			
Rule Out Choices			
A	B	C	D

44. The PN is administering a dose of methadone to a client. What actions should the PN take? (Select all that apply.)
   A. Determine the client's pain rating before giving the medication.
   B. Document that the medication was given directly after administration.
   C. Administer methadone on an empty stomach.
   D. Assess respiratory rate before and 1 hour after administration.
   E. Ask the client about his or her pain 30 to 60 minutes after administering.

HESI Test Question Approach				
Positive?			YES	NO
Key Words				
Rephrase				
Rule Out Choices				
A	B	C	D	E

45. The PN is working on a unit in an extended care facility. An 80-year-old male who is usually alert and oriented has become lethargic and his pulse rate is 128. What other findings would the PN look for in this client to confirm a possible urinary tract infection and early sepsis? (Select all that apply.)
   A. Increased respiratory rate
   B. Elevated temperature
   C. Cold, clammy skin
   D. New onset of incontinence
   E. Decreased blood pressure

HESI Test Question Approach				
Positive?			YES	NO
Key Words				
Rephrase				
Rule Out Choices				
A	B	C	D	E

46. The RN has indicated that a client is at high risk for falls. Which interventions should the PN expect to find in the plan of care to keep this client safe? (Select all that apply.)
    A. Slip-resistant socks applied
    B. Bed alarm turned on
    C. Side rails up × 4
    D. Urinary catheter in place
    E. Frequent checks

HESI Test Question Approach		
Positive?	YES	NO
Key Words		
Rephrase		
Rule Out Choices		
A B C D E		

47. A 3-year-old client is admitted for pneumonia. Ibuprofen 7.5 mg/kg every 6 hours is ordered. The child weighs 17.3 kg. The ibuprofen comes in a solution of 100 mg/5 mL. What is the ordered dose in milliliters for this child? (Answer in whole numbers.)

_____ mL

48. The PN is assisting with the admission of a client for observation after a motor vehicle accident. Which tasks can be safely assigned to the UAP? (Select all that apply.).
    A. Apply oxygen via nasal cannula to the client.
    B. Remove an IV from a painful, reddened IV site.
    C. Obtain a set of vital signs.
    D. Familiarize the client with the room.
    E. Clean the client's superficial wounds.

HESI Test Question Approach		
Positive?	YES	NO
Key Words		
Rephrase		
Rule Out Choices		
A B C D E		

49. A male client is newly diagnosed with heart failure. His wife asks the PN about the diet she should fix for her husband when he is discharged. What is the most effective technique to use to ensure that the wife understands?
    A. Provide appropriate handouts.
    B. Answer only the specific questions she asks.
    C. Use the teach-back method.
    D. Refer the wife to the dietician.

HESI Test Question Approach		
Positive?	YES	NO
Key Words		
Rephrase		
Rule Out Choices		
A B C D		

50. An elderly client is admitted who has a limited understanding of English. When reviewing instructions about his medications, which intervention should the PN implement?
   A. Wait for the translator to arrive.
   B. Use the son to translate.
   C. Provide written instructions.
   D. Use the video translation device.

HESI Test Question Approach			
Positive?		YES	NO
Key Words			
Rephrase			
Rule Out Choices			
A	B	C	D

51. While administering medications to a client, the PN hears the UAPs discussing another client in the hallway. Which intervention by the PN has highest priority?
   A. Inform the unit manager about the event.
   B. File an incident or occurrence report.
   C. Remind the UAPs about privacy requirements.
   D. Finish giving the medications.

HESI Test Question Approach			
Positive?		YES	NO
Key Words			
Rephrase			
Rule Out Choices			
A	B	C	D

ANSWERS AND RATIONALES

NOTE: Correct answers are underlined.

Management

1. Which activity should the practical nurse (PN) delegate to the unlicensed assistive personnel (UAP)? (Select all that apply.)

Rationales:

A. *Observe a client to see whether he or she can hear any better today after an IV antibiotic was discontinued (DC'd).*
This requires assessment about ototoxicity, which is beyond the scope of the UAP.

B. *Encourage additional PO fluids if an elderly client with pneumonia develops a fever.*
These directions are not sufficiently clear and detailed enough for the UAP to perform the task.

C. *Report the ability of a client to eat the food on the supper tray unassisted.*
This requires assessment of the client's clinical status that is beyond the scope of the UAP.

D. <u>*Record the number of liquid stools of a client who has received lactulose.*</u>
This is a task that encompasses basic care, elimination, and intake and output; it does not require judgment or the expertise of the nurse. It can be performed by the UAP.

E. <u>*Take the vital signs of clients scheduled for early morning tests.*</u>
This is a task that can easily be performed by the UAP and does not require interpretation of data.

2. The PN is caring for a group of clients with the assistance of several UAPs. Which situation requires an intervention by the PN?

Rationales:

A. *The client with active tuberculosis who is leaving his room without a mask.*
A UAP can be delegated to provide a box of masks or to direct the client back to his room.

B. *The client with pneumonia and dehydration who has not had anything to drink for 4 hours.*
A UAP can be directed to provide specific types and amounts of fluids.

C. <u>*The client with asthma who complains of being anxious and unable to concentrate.*</u>
This client is at risk for airway compromise and requires assessment. The PN should respond to this client.

D. *The client who is a high fall risk and is trying to get up to go to the bathroom.*
The UAP can assist the patient to the bathroom.

3. The PN reports that a hospitalized client has threatened to cut herself. In what order should the PN implement the following actions? (Place them in order, first to last.)
Answer: C, A, B, D
First: C. Stay with the client until a UAP is assigned to sit with client.
In order to keep the client safe, the first priority is to not leave the client alone.
Second: A. Perform a sweep of the room and remove any cords or sharp objects.
Even with a person in the room, a client may be able to use equipment in the room to harm himself or herself. Removing cords and sharp objects assists in keeping the client safe.
Third: B. Call the charge nurse and ask for an additional UAP.
It is not the best use of the PN's skills to remain in the room. This is a task that can be assigned to a UAP.
Fourth: D. Continue to establish rapport and ensure confidentiality.
Building rapport is important, but this client is a suicide risk; building rapport at this time and ensuring confidentiality will not ensure the client's safety, which is the priority.

4. The UAP is assisting with the care of several clients on a postpartum unit. Which assignment should the PN delegate to the UAP?

Rationales:

A. *Assess fundal firmness and lochia for the clients who delivered vaginally.*
Assessment is one of the roles of the nurse and is not consistent with the role of the UAP.

B. *Take vital signs every 15 minutes for a client with preeclampsia.*
This is a high-risk client who needs to be evaluated by a licensed nurse.

C. *Provide breast-feeding instructions for a primigravida.*
Teaching is also the responsibility of a licensed nurse.

D. <u>*Assist with daily care activities for all clients on bed rest.*</u>
This is the most appropriate assignment for the UAP. The PN should delegate daily care activities to the UAP based on the client's needs.

Advanced Clinical Concepts

5. Which client is at the highest risk for developing respiratory complications?

Rationales:

A. <u>*A 21-year-old with dehydration and cerebral palsy who is dependent in daily activities.*</u>
A client with dehydration and cerebral palsy (characterized by uncoordinated and spastic muscle movements that can cause ADL dependence) is at an increased risk for respiratory problems because of impaired mobility and swallowing.

B. *A 60-year-old who has had type 2 diabetes for 20 years and was admitted with cellulitis of the left leg.*

This client is more at risk for renal, cardiac, and/or vascular complications.

C. *An obese 30-year-old with hypertension who is noncompliant with the medication regimen.*

An obese individual who is noncompliant with antihypertensive meds is more at risk for cardiac or cerebral events than respiratory problems.

D. *A 40-year-old with a serum K^+ of 3.4 mEq/L, who is taking a loop diuretic and complains of fatigue.*

This middle-aged adult is hypokalemic and fatigued but is not at high risk for respiratory problems.

6. A PN is administering medications to a client with a history of substance abuse admitted for an overdose. Which interventions are priorities to include in this client's plan of care? (Select all that apply.)

A. *Allow the client to take his or her medications independently.*

This is not appropriate for a client who has recently taken an overdose.

B. *Ensure that all medications have been swallowed before leaving the client's room.*

With the client's history and reason for current admission, this ensures that the client is not saving medications to inappropriately take later.

C. *Request that oral pain medications be changed from tablet to oral suspension.*

Clients can try to hide tablets for ingestion or inhalation at a later time. By changing the dose to a liquid form, the nurse is making it more difficult for the patient to hide the medication.

D. *Give flumazemil every 6 hours around the clock.*

Flumazemil is used to reverse benzodiazepine overdose and is only given as needed.

E. *Only give medications to the client via the intravenous route.*

This is unnecessary and may contribute to the client's pattern of substance abuse.

7. A postoperative client has received normal saline intravenously at 125 mL/hr. The PN observes a dark yellow urine output. The first hour the output was 50 mL; the next hour, it was 32 mL; and the third hour, it was 28 mL. What action should the PN take?

Rationales:

A. *Give a bolus of D_5 ½ NS at 200 mL/hr.*

This is not a recommended action because hypertonic solutions are prescribed for fluid and electrolyte imbalances and cause an osmotic movement of fluids into the vasculature.

B. *Inform the registered nurse.*

Low urinary output may be a serious problem and requires more immediate intervention.

C. *Monitor output for another 2 hours.*

Urine output has been monitored and may indicate dehydration, which can lead to serious complications.

D. *Draw samples for BUN and creatinine labs.*

BUN and creatinine should be evaluated, but this is not the immediate priority.

8. A 54-year-old male client was admitted to the medical/surgical unit after a stapling of his esophageal varices. What intervention should the PN expect to be a part of this client's plan of care?

A. *Frequent oral suctioning*

Oral suctioning is not needed and may be harmful for this client.

B. *Bleeding precautions*

The client has cirrhosis of the liver and is prone to bleeding. These precautions, which include avoiding IM injections and holding pressure for a longer period for all venipunctures, are appropriate for this client.

C. *Diet high in protein*

Clients with cirrhosis of the liver need a diet low in protein.

D. *Complete bed rest*

Activity is encouraged for most clients. The client should be instructed to avoid activities that may cause bruising.

9. A client's arterial blood gas results are pH 7.29, P_{CO_2} 55 mm Hg, and HCO_3 26 mEq/L. Which is the correct interpretation of these values?

Rationales:

A. *Normal blood gas values*

Normal arterial blood gas values are: pH 7.35 to 7.45, P_{CO_2} 35 to 45 mm HG, and HCO_3 22 to 26 mEq/L.

B. *Respiratory acidosis*

The client's P_{CO_2} is 55, which demonstrates CO_2 retention and hypoventilation. The pH of 7.29 reflects acidosis with no compensation; therefore, it is respiratory acidosis.

C. *Respiratory alkalosis*

Typically ABG values indicating respiratory alkalosis include an increased pH value and a decrease in the P_{CO_2} due to hyperventilation.

D. *Metabolic acidosis*

ABG values indicating metabolic acidosis include a decreased pH value with a decrease in HCO_3 that occurs in such disorders as diabetic ketoacidosis and some types of kidney failure.

10. A client who has chronic back pain is not receiving adequate pain relief from an oral analgesic. What alternative action should the PN explore to promote the client's independence?

Rationales:
A. *Encourage the client to take the maximum dosage.*
Although this intervention may improve pain relief, it may not promote self-care without increasing side effects that may affect the client's independence.
B. *Obtain a prescription for an adjuvant medication.*
The addition of a second medication does not promote self-care and may cause additional side effects that interfere with the client's independence in ADLs.
C. *Consider the client's receptivity to using complementary therapy.*
This action supports increased pain control and self-care without the level of adverse effects associated with additional medication. It is the least invasive measure and promotes the active participation (self-care) of the client.
D. *Encourage counseling to prevent future addiction.*
Referrals may be necessary; however, it is the PN's responsibility to intervene with measures to manage pain and maintain self-care.

Maternal-Newborn Nursing

11. A client at 41 weeks' gestation who is in active labor calls the PN to report that her membranes have ruptured. The PN views the perineum and sees the cord. Which action should the PN implement first?

Rationales:
A. *Place the client in a knee-chest position.*
This is the most critical intervention to prevent cord compression by the presenting part, which would impair fetal oxygenation and lead to both morbidity and mortality.
B. *Cover the cord with sterile, warm NS gauze.*
If the cord is protruding outside the vagina, this should be done to prevent drying of the Wharton jelly; however, it is not the priority intervention.
C. *Assist with preparing for an emergency cesarean birth.*
This should be done by the staff while the client is kept in position to maintain the presenting part of the cord.
D. *Start oxygen by face mask at 10 L/min.*
Oxygen should be provided to the mother to increase oxygen to the fetus via the placenta; however, the priority is to maintain the presenting part of the cord.

12. A client at 39 weeks' gestation plans to have an epidural block when labor is established. What intervention(s) should the PN implement to prevent side effects?

Rationales:
A. *Reinforce teaching about the procedure and the effects of the epidural.*
Teaching the client about the procedure and the expected results of epidural analgesia is an important nursing intervention; however, it does not prevent the side effects.
B. *Place the client in a chair next to the bed with her feet elevated.*
An epidural block reduces lower extremity sensation and movement to varying degrees. Positions such as sitting in a chair may not be possible during epidural pain management; also, they may be a safety risk and may not prevent side effects.
C. *Monitor the fetal heart rate and contractions continuously.*
Vital signs should be monitored every 5 minutes immediately after the initial epidural dose, and if stable, then every 15 minutes.
D. *Assist the client to empty her bladder every 2 hours.*
Because the client may be unable to determine whether she has a full bladder, assisting her to void every 2 hours prevents urinary retention, a side effect of epidural anesthesia.

13. A client whose last menses was 6 weeks ago presents in the clinic with right lower quadrant abdominal pain, no vaginal bleeding, and pain in her right shoulder. Which action should the PN take first?

Rationales:
A. *Check for abdominal rebound tenderness, distention, and fever.*
Bleeding related to an ectopic pregnancy may present these manifestations, but first the PN should assess for hypovolemic shock.
B. *Obtain vital signs and assist with IV access.*
The PN should first evaluate the client's vital signs for indications of shock related to a ruptured ectopic pregnancy (an obstetric emergency). A vascular access is vital if shock should occur.
C. *Observe for recent musculoskeletal injury, bruising, or abuse.*
This may be part of the assessment if a life-threatening situation is ruled out first.
D. *Collect specimens for a pregnancy test, hemoglobin level, and WBC count.*
A pregnancy test and blood work is needed, but first the PN should collect further data to determine if the client is showing signs of shock secondary to intraabdominal bleeding.

14. A pregnant client with a low hematocrit and low hemoglobin asks the PN why she should take her iron supplement. Which explanation should the PN offer?

Rationales:

A. *Iron promotes collagen production, which aids healing during the postpartum period.*
This does not explain the need for the additional iron.

B. *Iron reduces the risk of preterm labor.*
This does not explain the need for the additional iron.

C. *Replacing iron through the diet alone is difficult.*
With the expansion of plasma volume and the use of iron by the fetus to build hemoglobin, pregnant women have difficulty replacing iron losses through nutrition alone.

D. *Additional iron will be necessary to replace blood loss during delivery.*
This does not explain the need for the additional iron during the pregnancy.

Medical-Surgical Review

15. A client is returning to the unit after an intravenous pyelogram (IVP). Which intervention should the PN include in the plan of care?

Rationales:

A. *Maintain bed rest.*
There is no need to restrict mobility after an IVP.

B. *Increase fluid intake.*
The client should increase PO fluids to facilitate excretion of the dye, thereby preventing possible side effects.

C. *Monitor for hematuria.*
There is no risk of hematuria from an IVP.

D. *Continue NPO status.*
The client should resume fluid intake after an IVP to facilitate excretion of the dye.

16. A female client has chronic urinary tract infections. The PN is reinforcing teaching to the client about a prescription for ciprofloxacin 500 mg PO bid. What side effect(s) could the client expect over the course of medication therapy? (Select all that apply.)

Rationales:

A. *Photosensitivity*
This is a side effect of ciprofloxacin; exposure to sunlight or tanning beds should be avoided. The client should be instructed to use sunscreen and to wear protective clothing.

B. *Dyspepsia*
Ciprofloxacin causes GI irritation, nausea and vomiting, and abdominal pain, which should be reported.

C. *Diarrhea*
Watery, foul-smelling diarrhea is an adverse reaction to ciprofloxacin and an indicator of pseudomembranous colitis; this must be reported and requires immediate intervention.

D. *Urinary frequency*
Although not a side effect of ciprofloxacin, urinary frequency may indicate that the medication is ineffective and should be reported.

E. *Anemia*
This is not an expected side effect of ciprofloxacin.

17. A PN working on a hospice unit finds a client crying. The client states that he is afraid to die. Which actions should the PN implement? (Select all that apply).

A. *Sit quietly with the client and listen to his concerns.*
Silence, or offering one's presence, is an effective technique that lets the client share as he desires and also shows that the nurse cares.

B. *Provide the client with privacy.*
The client has shared that he is afraid. Further isolating the client from others will not address this need.

C. *Administer an antianxiety medication to the client.*
The nurse may eventually decide to give the client a medication to help with his anxiety, but this should not be the first action.

D. *Ask client's permission to contact a spiritual counselor or minister.*
Facing death is a spiritual issue. Requesting help from the client's spiritual provider is appropriate.

E. *Assess the patient for signs of impending death.*
The client is awake and oriented. There is no indication that the client's death is imminent.

18. A client with a peritoneal dialysis catheter calls the clinic to report that he feels poorly and seems to have a fever. What is the PN's best response?

Rationales:

A. *Encourage the client to come to the clinic today to be evaluated.*
The catheter places the client at risk for a peritoneal infection. Because clients receiving peritoneal dialysis usually have some degree of immune compromise and anemia, this client should come to the clinic to be assessed.

B. *Instruct the client to increase his fluid intake to 3 L/day.*
Clients who need dialysis retain fluid and usually are restricted to an intake that is only 300 mL greater than output.

C. *Review the client's peritoneal dialysis regimen.*
The nurse should evaluate the client's regimen; however, assessing the client for infection is a higher priority.

D. *Ask the client about his recent dietary intake of protein and iron.*
Iron deficiency and protein loss are common problems in clients who are receiving peritoneal dialysis. Although monitoring dietary intake is important, it does not take priority over evaluating for possible infection.

19. A client is admitted with chest pain. Which assessment finding(s) should be reported to the charge nurse immediately? (Select all that apply.)

Rationales:
A. *Diaphoresis*
   Clients experiencing a myocardial infarction (MI) are often diaphoretic.
B. *Irregular heart rate*
   Dysrhythmias are one of the most frequent complications of an MI.
C. *Elevated troponin level*
   Troponin I is cardiac specific and therefore a highly specific indicator of an MI.
D. *Radiating jaw pain*
   Pain is the foremost symptom of MI, and jaw pain is considered one of the classic signs.
E. *O$_2$ saturation of 93%*
   This is a normal finding.

20. The PN is reviewing the discharge instructions with a client who has a history of angina. Which instruction should the PN emphasize as the most important?

Rationales:
A. *Avoid activity that will require the Valsalva maneuver.*
   Although minimizing or avoiding the Valsalva maneuver decreases anginal pain, it is not the most important issue.
B. *Seek emergency treatment if chest pain persists after the third nitroglycerin dose.*
   This instruction is the most important because chest pain characteristic of acute myocardial infarction persists longer than 15 minutes and delaying medical treatment can be life threatening.
C. *Rest for 30 minutes after having chest pain before resuming activity.*
   Waiting 30 minutes may be recommended only if the nitroglycerin is effective.
D. *Keep extra nitroglycerin in an airtight, light-resistant bottle.*
   This is an excellent medication teaching point; however, it does not have the same urgency as seeking emergency care.

21. The PN is reviewing the medication diltiazem with a client. Which dietary recommendation should be included?

Rationales:
A. *Maintain a low-sodium diet.*
   The client may need to restrict the sodium intake, but that is not specific for diltiazem.
B. *Eat a banana each morning.*
   If the client has low potassium, this should be recommended; however, it is not the highest priority.

C. *Eat high-fiber foods daily.*
   This is an excellent teaching point for everyone, but it is not specific for diltiazem.
D. *Avoid grapefruit products.*
   Grapefruit should be avoided by clients taking calcium channel blockers because it can cause an increase in the medication's serum level, predisposing the client to hypotension.

22. A female client with a history of Raynaud's disease wants to know how to manage her symptoms. What teaching should the PN reinforce?

Rationales:
A. *Take oral analgesic at regularly spaced intervals.*
   Pain, unlike the feeling of cold hands and fingers, is not always associated with Raynaud's syndrome. If pain is present, it is sporadic and situational, which should not require continuous medication.
B. *Avoid extremes of heat and cold.*
   In Raynaud's syndrome, vascular spasms of the hands and fingers are triggered by extremes of heat or cold. The PN should encourage the client to avoid these triggers, which elicit pallor and cold-to-the-touch sensations.
C. *Limit intake of foods and fluids with caffeine.*
   Caffeine is not a primary trigger, but it should be limited if the client notes that it contributes to blanching.
D. *Keep involved extremities in a dependent position.*
   This is not effective for a client with Raynaud's syndrome.

23. The PN is providing care for a client admitted with thrombocytopenia. Which problem should the PN immediately report to the charge nurse?

Rationales:
A. *Bleeding gums*
   Bleeding gums are a sign of extremely low platelet count and should be reported.
B. *Refusing breakfast*
   Although a poor appetite may be a symptom of thrombocytopenia, reporting bleeding gums takes priority in the client with thrombocytopenia.
C. *Complaints of insomnia*
   Insomnia is not a typical symptom associated with thrombocytopenia and is not the priority problem at this time.
D. *Constant fatigue*
   This is a problem typically associated with a client who is anemic and there is no need for emergent intervention.

24. A client admitted with cancer of the larynx is scheduled for a laryngectomy tomorrow. What client education should the PN review with him tonight?

Rationales:
A. *Anticipated body image changes*
This is a common need and should be addressed after the diagnosis has been made, surgery has been performed, and basic needs and communication techniques have been met.
B. *Pain management expectations*
Pain management is important, but the ability to vocalize or convey these needs should be addressed first.
C. *Communication techniques*
The nurse should review communication techniques, making sure the client understands alternative ways to express and convey basic subjective needs in the immediate postoperative period.
D. *Postoperative nutritional needs*
Nutrition is important to promote healing, but the client should understand ways to communicate needs in the immediate postoperative period.

Mental Health Nursing

25. A victim of a motor vehicle collision is dead on arrival at the emergency department. Which action should the nurse take to assist the spouse?

Rationales:
A. *Ask whether there are relatives, friends, or clergy to call.*
The PN should help the spouse identify support systems and resources for coping.
B. *Talk about the former relationship with the spouse.*
The PN should focus on immediate needs for coping and support; the spouse may be unable to process information during the crisis.
C. *Provide education about the stages of grief and loss.*
The spouse is unable to focus on learning about grief and loss during the crisis.
D. *Assess the spouse's level of anxiety.*
Although the level of anxiety affects the client's response to the crisis, the PN should assist the client in coping with the present stressful event.

26. The PN is interviewing a client in the prenatal clinic about violence during pregnancy. Which statement (s) describe(s) an appropriate technique to assess for violence? (Select all that apply.)

Rationales:
A. *Women should be assessed only if they are part of high-risk groups.*
Violence against women occurs in all ethnic groups and at all income levels.

B. *Women may be assessed in the presence of young children.*
It is important that children not be present because they may repeat what is heard. Infants may be present.
C. *Women should be assessed only once during pregnancy.*
Many women do not reveal violence the first time they are asked. As trust develops between nurse and client, the client may be more comfortable sharing her story. Also, violence may start later in the pregnancy.
D. *Women should be reassessed face to face by a nurse as the pregnancy progresses.*
Having more than one face-to-face interview elicits the highest reports of violence during pregnancy.
E. *Women should be assessed alone, without the intimate partner.*
Interviewing the client in private allows her to be comfortable in sharing her story.

27. The PN reminds several clients on the mental health unit that breakfast is at 0800, medications are given at 0900, and group therapy sessions begin at 1000. Which treatment modality has been implemented?

Rationales:
A. *Milieu therapy*
Milieu therapy uses resources and activities in the environment to assist with improving social functioning and activities of daily living.
B. *Behavior modification*
Behavior modification involves changing behaviors with positive and negative reinforcements to allow desired activities or remove privileges.
C. *Peer therapy*
Peer therapy is not a single therapeutic modality, but peers are responsible for supporting, sharing, and compromising within their peer group and milieu.
D. *Problem-solving*
Problem-solving is related to crisis intervention where the nurse focuses on the problem and ways to reestablish previous levels of functioning.

28. The PN, who is taking a client to the radiography department, starts to enter the elevator with him. The client becomes panic-stricken and states, "I can't do this." Which intervention should the PN implement first?

Rationales:
A. *Ask one more staff member to ride in the elevator.*
One more staff member will not be able to assist the client to overcome his fears until he first can recognize his feelings.

B. *Offer an antianxiety medication.*
   Offering an antianxiety medication may be necessary to begin desensitization but is not the priority.
C. *Begin desensitization about riding the elevator.*
   Desensitizing the client may be implemented, but first the client should identify his fear and recognize his anxiety.
D. <u>*Affirm his fears about riding the elevator.*</u>
   The PN should first affirm the client's feelings of anxiety and fear about riding the elevator; then options for desensitization may be considered.

29. **A male client, who is suffering from posttraumatic stress disorder, is found one night trying to strangle his roommate. Which interventions should the PN implement immediately? (Select all that apply).**

Rationales:
   A. *Give the client a sedative.*
      A sedative may reduce anxiety and encourage sleep, but safety is the most important intervention.
   B. *Ask the victim to share his feelings.*
      Processing the trauma with the victim is important, but safety is the priority.
   C. <u>*Move the client to a private room.*</u>
      The PN should focus on safety as the immediate concern and move the client to a private room to protect both clients from harm.
   D. *Place the client in restraints.*
      Restraints should only be used when a client does not respond to verbal reminders.
   E. <u>*Assign a UAP to sit with the client.*</u>
      Clients who are at risk for hurting themselves or others should not be left alone.

30. **The PN is providing care for a client with a borderline personality disorder who is being manipulative. Which intervention should the PN expect to see in the client's plan of care?**

Rationales:
   A. <u>*Refer the client's requests to one nurse.*</u>
      The best intervention is to provide consistency and avoid splitting by assigning the client to only one nurse.
   B. *Do not challenge inappropriate behavior.*
      The PN should assist the client in recognizing manipulative behavior and set limits on manipulative behaviors as needed.
   C. *Limit the client's contacts with other clients.*
      Socialization should be encouraged to improve skills with others.
   D. *Remove consequences for acting-out behavior.*
      Firm limits with clear expectations and consequences are necessary for clients who are manipulative.

31. **An adolescent client, admitted to the mental health unit for anorexia nervosa, frequently isolates herself. What is the PN's priority intervention?**

Rationales:
   A. *Teach the client the importance of self-expression.*
      Self-expression of feelings is important, but re-establishing eating habits is the priority intervention.
   B. <u>*Monitor the client's activities closely.*</u>
      The PN should monitor and supervise the client's activities to prevent bingeing, purging, or avoiding meals.
   C. *Include the client in daily group therapy.*
      The client should be included in daily groups, but the priority is her physiological needs, including monitoring meals.
   D. *Facilitate social interactions with others.*
      The client should be given opportunities to socialize, but monitoring activities during the day, especially meals, is the priority.

32. **The PN is planning the daily schedule for clients on the mental health unit. A male client who is manic should be encouraged to participate in which group activity?**

Rationales:
   A. *A basketball game in the gym*
      The client should avoid any potentially competitive physical activity; basketball is a contact sport that may stimulate aggressive acting-out behavior.
   B. <u>*Jogging at least 1 mile*</u>
      Jogging is the best activity for this client because it is a noncompetitive physical activity that expends the energy associated with mania.
   C. *A Ping-Pong game with a peer*
      The PN should avoid assigning the client to competitive activities that can cause frustration and stimulate mood swings.
   D. *A group activity with the art therapist*
      A manic client may become disruptive and distracted in an art group; also, physical energy using large muscle groups is more effective for expending energy.

Delegation and Prioritization

33. **A PN is making client assignments for the night shift. The nursing team has another PN and two UAPs. Which duties could be delegated to the UAPs? (Select all that apply.)**

Rationales:
   A. <u>*Transport a client who has had a stroke to the radiology department for a chest radiograph.*</u>

UAPs may obtain vital signs and weight and height measurements, perform care activities, transport clients, and do secretarial work. The PN should instruct the UAP in the proper precautions for these delegated procedures as needed.

B. *Reinforce the technique for injecting insulin to a client newly diagnosed with diabetes.*
The ability to reinforce teaching requires the critical thinking and knowledge application skills unique to the licensed nurse.

C. *Bathe a 25-year-old client who is a quadriplegic and has a large, stage IV pressure ulcer.*
The UAP may obtain vital signs and weight and height measurements, perform care activities, transport clients, and do secretarial work. The PN should instruct the UAP on proper precautions for these delegated procedures as needed.

D. *Turn a 92-year-old end-stage heart failure client who is a DNR.*
UAPs may obtain vital signs and weight and height measurements, perform care activities, transport clients, and do secretarial work. The PN should instruct the UAP in the proper precautions for these delegated procedures as needed.

E. *Inform family members that visiting hours are over.*
UAPs may obtain vital signs and weight and height measurements, perform care activities, transport clients, and do secretarial work. The PN should instruct the UAP in the proper precautions for these delegated procedures as needed.

34. A hospitalized client has type 2 diabetes. Which task(s) for this client can the PN delegate to the UAP? (Select all that apply.)

Rationales:

A. *Notifying the dietitian of a prescribed consult.*
The UAP may perform simple secretarial tasks.

B. *Reporting the client's insulin injection technique.*
The ability to reinforce teaching requires the critical thinking and knowledge application skills unique to the licensed nurse.

C. *Obtaining the finger stick blood glucose level before meals.*
The UAP may obtain finger stick blood glucose levels.

D. *Reminding the client to dry the toes carefully after a shower.*
Hygiene tasks may be delegated to the UAP.

E. *Talking with the client about foods that raise the blood glucose level.*
The ability to reinforce teaching requires the critical thinking and knowledge application skills unique to the licensed nurse.

35. After change-of-shift report, the PN reviews her assignments. Which client should the PN assess first?

Rationales:

A. *The elderly client receiving palliative care for heart failure who complains of constipation and nervousness.*
Constipation and nervousness are concerns, but these are common problems in palliative care; this is not the priority client.

B. *A client who is admitted with possible pneumonia with a heart rate of 110 and a respiratory rate of 24.*
Tachycardia and tachypnea are two of the SIRS criteria, signs of early sepsis. This client needs to be seen first.

C. *A middle-aged client with end-stage renal failure whose urinary output was 95 mL for 8 hours.*
Oliguria or anuria is an expected outcome in chronic renal failure; this is not the priority client.

D. *A client taking Coumadin who is receiving oxygen at 3 L/min and has respirations of 12 breaths/min.*
A respiratory rate of 12 breaths/min is an acceptable vital sign; this is not the priority client.

36. The female PN has been assigned to care for a male Muslim client who has a recent ostomy. Which actions would demonstrate cultural sensitivity? (Select all that apply.)

A. *Cover her hair with a cloth when going into the patient's room.*
This is not expected by the client and may be even considered offensive.

B. *Ask a male UAP to assist the client with his bath.*
Clients of the Muslim faith are modest and prefer having a person of the same sex assist with their bath.

C. *Move the bed to face the east.*
Practicing Muslims pray five times during the day and try to face Mecca (which is to the east) when they pray. Placing the bed in an east-facing direction facilitates this practice.

D. *Ensure that there is no pork in his food.*
Pork is prohibited in the Muslim diet.

E. *Provide the client with a new ostomy bag before each prayer time.*
Before prayer, the Muslim believer will do a ceremonial washing. At this time, if they have an ostomy, they will also want to have a clean bag.

37. The PN enters the exam room after a client has been told by her healthcare provider that she has advanced ovarian cancer. Which response by the nurse is likely to be most supportive for the client?

Rationales:

A. *Share with the client information about survivor rates.*
Providing information does not allow the client to process her feelings.

B. *Discuss with the client the different treatment options.*
Providing facts does not allow the client to process her feelings.

C. *Encourage the client to get a second opinion.*
Providing an opinion does not allow the client to process her feelings.

D. *Sit quietly with the client and allow her to express her feelings.*
This allows the client to decide on the communication; if the PN is directing and talking, the goals of therapeutic communication are thwarted.

38. **Which assessment finding indicates the expected outcome of administering donepezil to a client with Alzheimer's disease?**

Rationales:

A. *Increased muscle strength and tone*
Aricept does not improve muscle strength.

B. *Fewer episodes of urinary incontinence*
Aricept does not improve continence.

C. *Increased ability to solve simple problems*
Aricept is used for mild to moderate Alzheimer's disease and helps improve cognitive function.

D. *Improved appetite, supporting weight gain*
Aricept does not improve appetite.

39. **In caring for an older client with sundowning syndrome, which intervention(s) should the PN implement? (Select all that apply.)**

Rationales:

A. *Observe for tiredness at the end of the day.*
Monitoring the client for tiredness is important because these signs may affect sundowning syndrome.

B. *Maintain a quiet unit during the late afternoon.*
Noise levels can affect the client's orientation level. A noisy environment may increase agitation as the day progresses.

C. *Monitor for medication side effects.*
Monitoring the client for side effects is important because these may affect sundowning syndrome.

D. *Assess for decreased gross motor movement.*
This is not an expected finding with sundowning syndrome.

E. *Reorient the client to reality.*
Reality orientation does not work in the client with dementia and often increases agitation.

40. **When the PN begins to assist an elderly male client with dementia to get out of bed, the client becomes angry and yells at the nurse, "Get out of here! I'll get up when I'm ready." Which action by the nurse is most likely to be helpful in reducing the client's agitation?**

Rationales:

A. *Continue to encourage the client to get out of bed.*
This action would likely continue to agitate the client.

B. *Explain why ambulation is important.*
Providing information to a client who cannot process his or her behavior only increases the client's agitation.

C. *Acknowledge how he feels but continue to get him out of bed.*
Providing information to a client who cannot process his or her behavior only increases the client's agitation.

D. *Return in 30 minutes and try again.*
Clients with dementia are unable to reflect on their unacceptable behavior and learn to control it. Therefore, providing a time-out away from the nurse is the correct response. The client needs the time and space to de-escalate.

41. **A client with diabetes is admitted for osteomyelitis. Which regimen for hypoglycemic control would the PN expect the healthcare provider to prescribe for this client?**

A. *Supplemental scale using regular insulin*
This therapy is designed to correct hyperglycemia after it has occurred. It is not the best option.

B. *Continue home oral hypoglycemic medications*
Oral agents should be discontinued during acute illness and whenever oral intake may be inconsistent.

C. *An alpha-glucosidase inhibitor*
Alpha-glucosidase inhibitors should not be used when there is any possibility of the need of iodinated contrast studies.

D. *A combination of long-acting and short-acting insulin*
Scheduled basal/bolus insulin is designed to prevent hyperglycemia and is the best option for inpatient glycemic control.

42. **The PN is making a home visit to provide wound care for an 80-year-old man. The PN suspects that the client is being physically abused. Which intervention should the PN implement first?**

A. *Notify the RN case manager.*
The registered nurse needs to do an assessment and validate the findings before it is reported to authorities.

B. *Confront the caregiver.*
Confrontation is not appropriate and could escalate the situation.

C. *Call the police.*
   This may be needed if the client is in imminent danger, but first the RN needs to complete an assessment.
D. *Ask the client to validate the abuse.*
   Many elderly clients deny that the abuse occurs. This may not provide any additional information.

43. **The PN is working on a hospice unit. A client is resting quietly but moans when turned. The family has asked the nurse for more pain medication for the client. How should the PN respond?**
   A. *Discuss with the family why they believe the client needs more pain medication.*
      Having an open discussion with the family may help decrease their concerns that the client is in pain and help them to understand the balance between oversedation and keeping the client comfortable.
   B. *Ask the family to leave to allow the client to rest.*
      In end-of-life care, a key component of care is to allow the family to remain at the bedside as much as possible.
   C. *Since the client is in hospice care, give the medication as the family requests.*
      It is the nurse's responsibility, not the family's, to assess if the client needs pain medication.
   D. *Ask the charge nurse to request a prescription for a sedative for the client.*
      The client is resting comfortably, a sedative is not needed.

44. **The PN is administering a dose of methadone. What actions should the PN take? (Select all that apply.)**
   A. *Determine the client's pain rating before giving the medication.*
      Before administering a pain medication, the client's pain should be assessed, which includes rating how severe the pain is.
   B. *Document that the medication was given directly after administration.*
      Accurate and timely documentation is an essential aspect of medication administration.
   C. *Administer methadone on an empty stomach.*
      Some clients tolerate methadone better when there is food in the stomach.
   D. *Assess respiratory rate before and 1 hour after administration.*
      Methadone is a synthetic opioid and can cause respiratory depression.
   E. *Ask the client about his or her pain 30 to 60 minutes after administering.*
      Reassessing the client's pain 30 to 60 minutes after administration is necessary to determine the effectiveness of the medication.

45. **The PN is working on a unit in an extended care facility. An 80-year-old male who is usually alert and oriented has become lethargic and his pulse rate is 128. What other findings would the PN look for in this client to confirm a possible urinary tract infection and early sepsis? (Select all that apply.)**
   A. *Increased respiratory rate*
      With an infection, the respiratory rate often increases along with an increase in pulse and temperature.
   B. *Elevated temperature*
      An elevated temperature is a cardinal sign that an infectious process is occurring.
   C. *Cold, clammy skin*
      Cold, clammy skin is more a sign of shock than a sign of an infection.
   D. *New onset of incontinence*
      For the elderly, an early sign of a urinary tract infection is that a client who was continent becomes incontinent.
   E. *Decreased blood pressure*
      With infections, damaged endothelium increases capillary permeability, allowing fluid to leak into body tissues, resulting in hypotension.

46. **The RN has indicated that a client is at high risk for falls. Which interventions should the PN expect to find in the plan of care to keep this client safe? (Select all that apply.)**
   A. *Slip-resistant socks applied*
      Slip-resistant socks help prevent the client from sliding when the client is ambulating.
   B. *Bed alarm turned on*
      Clients at high risk for falls should have an active bed alarm to remind the client to ask for help when getting out of bed and to alert the staff that the client is trying to get up.
   C. *Side rails up × 4*
      All four side rails being up is considered a restraint and actually might contribute to a fall if the client attempts to climb over them to get out of bed.
   D. *Urinary catheter in place*
      Urinary catheters actually increase rather than decrease the risk for falling.
   E. *Frequent checks*
      Frequently checking on the client and asking about the need to use the toilet or if the client has other needs may prevent the client from getting up without assistance and prevent a fall.

47. **A 3-year-old client is admitted for pneumonia. Ibuprofen 7.5 mg/kg every 6 hours is ordered. The child weighs 17.3 kg. The ibuprofen comes in a solution of 100 mg/5 mL. What is the ordered dose in milliliters for this child? (Answer in whole numbers.)**

   $$7.5 \text{ mg/kg} \times 17.3 \text{ kg} = 129.8 \text{ mg}$$
   $$130 \text{ mg} \times 5 \text{ mL}/100 \text{ mg} = 6.5 \text{ mL}$$

   Should rounding be necessary, it is to be performed at the end of the calculation.

48. The PN is assisting with the admission of a client for observation after a motor vehicle accident. Which tasks can be safely assigned to the UAP? (Select all that apply.)
   A. *Apply oxygen via nasal cannula to the client.*
      Oxygen is a medication. A nurse needs to initiate oxygen.
   B. *Remove an IV from a painful, reddened IV site.*
      The site needs to be evaluated for the need for further treatment. This is a nursing responsibility.
   C. *Obtain a set of vital signs.*
      This is a task that is commonly performed by the UAP.
   D. *Familiarize the client with the room.*
      This task does not require special training and can be assigned to the UAP.
   E. *Clean the client's superficial wounds.*
      Assessment and documentation of all wounds need to be completed by the nurse.

49. A male client is newly diagnosed with heart failure. His wife asks the PN about the diet she should fix for her husband when he is discharged. What is the most effective technique to use to ensure that the wife understands?
   A. *Provide appropriate handouts.*
      The use of handouts does not give the nurse any indication that the client's wife understands the client's diet.
   B. *Answer only the specific questions she asks.*
      Answering the wife's questions does allow her to direct the conversation, but it does not indicate what she understands.
   C. *Use the teach-back method.*
      The teach-back method is one of the best methods to use to ensure that the wife understands the instructions given. Patient understanding is confirmed when the wife can explain what the nurse has taught.
   D. *Refer the wife to the dietician.*
      The dietician would be an excellent source of information for the wife about her husband's diet, but again, it does not assess what the client's wife understands.

50. An elderly client is admitted who has a limited understanding of English. When reviewing instructions about his medications, which intervention should the PN implement?
   A. *Wait for the translator to arrive.*
      Having a translator at the bedside is ideal. Since this is review of his medications and not a crucial conversation (such as obtaining consent for surgery), other less costly options can be considered.
   B. *Use the son to translate.*
      Best practices discourage healthcare personnel from using family members as translators.
   C. *Provide written instructions.*
      While instructions written in the client's native language may be helpful, this is not the best answer.
   D. *Use the video translation device.*
      These allow the translator to see and interact with both the client and the PN while avoiding the expense of having the translator travel to the facility.

51. While administering medications to a client, the PN hears the UAPs discussing another client in the hallway. Which intervention by the PN has highest priority?
   A. *Inform the unit manager about the event.*
      The PN should inform the unit manager about the event, but this is not the first action to take.
   B. *File an incident or occurrence report.*
      Depending on the facility's policies, the PN may need to fill out a report, but this is not the first priority.
   C. *Remind the UAPs about privacy requirements.*
      The PN needs to stop the inappropriate conversation. This is the highest priority and essential to maintaining the client's privacy.
   D. *Finish giving the medications.*
      The PN can return to the administration of medications after stopping the inappropriate actions by the UAPs.